To Angie

Thirty-Ei
Li

anne xx

A Selection of Empowering and Inspirational Essays for Personal Growth, Overcoming Adversity and Finding Happiness

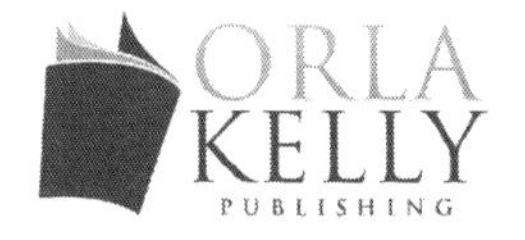

ANNE WATSON

978-1-914225-00-0

Published in Ireland by Orla Kelly Publishing. Edited by Red Pen Edits.

To my family and friends especially Larry. Thanks to all for being there when it mattered the most.

Acknowledgements

Thanks to Hilda Simpson and Brian Grimes for the encouragement to put these 38 articles into a book. Thanks also to Orla Kelly and Jean O'Sullivan for making the book a reality.

About the Author

Anne is a teacher who writes in her spare time. Anne is very interested in the self-development and growth of people. The articles were written randomly over time for readers who find themselves reflecting on life, habits, thoughts and actions like Anne herself often did.

Something would happen to Anne and she found herself reflecting on the experience to try and find a way to develop and grow as a person and create a positive outcome. So that the next time something similar would happen Anne and her readers would be aware of the outcome turning the outcome into something positive and enlightening. This is the aim of the book to help people in similar situations having similar experiences to learn from obstacles and barriers in their daily lives and overcome them. That once the reader has read some of the articles that he/she would feel better or lighter in him/herself.

Contents

CHAPTER 1

A new reality

Can we now, like never before, create a new global reality where we all live on this magnificent blue planet together in peace and harmony? Can we now learn to balance the scales of life in favour for us all to flourish and bloom like it is meant to be in the beginning? Can we now all learn to balance and share in a global good fortune and a global fountain of abundance for each one of us? Why has this never happened before?

The reason is that a global abundance mindset did not have the majority.

Now we do.

This pandemic has now, once and for all, taught us to put health before wealth. The governments of the world are standing up for us all. Once we have won the battle to curb the pandemic, we can create a longer lasting future for each one of us and future generations to come.

The scales of humanity will be in balance once and for all. We will all share a positive productive mindset in favour of a better world. Each individual will walk the path of his/her destiny and be who they are meant to be. We will never again have to walk alone. We will have all we need to fulfil our purpose and destiny. We will never have to carry chains of slavery in any shape or form again. Previously the scales became unbalanced in favour of the 'have' as opposed to the 'have nots', those with wealth and those without wealth. The purgatory of chains crisscrossed our lives, minds, hearts and souls.

But we know too that wealth carries its own punishments as well as not having enough to live on does. Wealth's punishments include the illusion of happiness. The Judas kiss of betrayal that puts money before loyalty, sincerity, truth, friendship. Living in the coldness of their big houses with not enough love, kindness, gentleness to fill the rooms. All you can find in these large soulless bare houses belongs to the old world of greed, selfishness and emptiness along with the fear of not having enough.

But the 'have nots' also have a share in this out of balance world as they too tried to climb the ladder of the wealthy and tried to become like them by stepping on all those who got in the way. The whole source of the problem comes down to an unbalanced, poverty riddled mindset.

If we change our mindset to see the world as not our property but to see it as something to share and pass on to the next generation, we can therefore change from a poverty consciousness to an abundant consciousness. When we all realise that we own nothing, that we cannot bring anything with us, that we can only pass our resources on to those we leave behind, we will understand and learn the correct mindset for peace and harmony in this magnificent world of ours.

We will learn that a global mindset fixed on helping us all is really the gold dust we have all being searching for. That mindset is within our grasps if we can learn to share and give out what we have, instead of hoarding and emasculating huge resources for the few and for banks to learn to forgo their policy of debt and desire to ensnare us in their chains of the nightmare of never ever going to be able to pay them back as the resources are limited in the first place. Money has no value. But people have value and are the best innovative resource we will ever have. It is people we need to buy into, not money.

Until now it was financial, mental, emotional or spiritual enslavement we have all been embroiled in. We were all swimming in this soup of knots of what we can't do instead of what we can do. The mindset of the rich and powerful was to enslave and stay superior of the minority. The desire was to control those of us who understood the correct mindset but did not have the resources to overcome the obstacles that were placed in front of us every day.

The system favoured the rich – that is nothing new to most of us. But now we have the possibility with the present pandemic to lift the crown of chains the rich and powerful have placed around us. It looks like they will carry their own crown of metal thorns as their wealth no longer has the value it had before because now our global health is more important than our national wealth.

Governments throughout the world are putting health before wealth. People's lives now have more value than how much money is in their account. This is nothing short of miraculous. No longer will we need to look to the past as we have now a mindset where people come first and their resources second. That the person lying in a hospital bed is no different to the person lying in the other. Both are entitled to the same level of care because of the actions taken by our governments.

The virus does not differentiate nor will our new mindset when this pandemic is under control. The government is protecting us all by putting all the necessary resources in place to protect us, such as preparing hospitals, movement restrictions, closing schools, providing funding to all self-employed – no one is being left out. This level of political care is unprecedented in our history and it is being shown by governments globally.

The world will never be the same again. The time has come for all of us to stand together equally with one true, positive productive mindset to stand shoulder to shoulder as it was meant to be.

We will win the day and peace and harmony will reign at it was meant to be.

CHAPTER 2

Approval junkie

Do you spend your time thinking about what others think?

Do you spend your time stressing over how you look?

Do you spend your time keeping up with your friends?

Do you spend time trying to fit in?

Then you are depending on others, chained to their opinions, chained to their emotions and living an emotionally reactive life. All of this, just to get their ever-invaluable approval?

Did you know that by seeking others approval, we give away our power and self-worth? We are giving out signals that we are inferior and need someone else to make us feel better. The outcome of being an approval junkie is that we live a life on a rollercoaster, going from one emotional fix to another, ranging from big highs to devastating lows. One minute we are up and feeling great, with just a word from someone else we are on the downward slope again to pain.

We become a ravaged addict, a victim, and an emotional wreck seeking the ultimate high of approval. We become what is known as a behavioural addict, forever increasing our dosage to get that original kick. But then the big crash happens. We come down. But we want to be up and so the chain starts again. We seek out that illusive buzz of approval again and again, on and on the vicious cycle repeats and repeats itself. The problem is the bigger the craving gets, the more dependent we become on others to change our mood and give us that kick.

To help ourselves, we have to withdraw from the need to be re-injected all the time with someone else's approval. We have to heal our cravings like a drug addict needs to heal his/her cravings from drug/substance dependency. We need to release our dependencies on our partner, family, friends, and work colleagues. We need to learn how to improve our own mood with meditation, exercise, and new hobbies. We need to learn to avoid dipping into the abyss of negativity, which leads us to search for a quick fix of approval from others.

We need to build up our own self-worth. We need to let go of depending on people to make us feel good. Everyone has the power to make himself or herself happy and have inner peace inside without looking for it from anyone else. No one has the right to dictate to another person how he or she should feel, how he or she should think, and how he or she should react. Other people should not have any power over our moods and emotions. Only we ourselves can decide how we feel at any one moment and no one else.

We all need to have a healthy amount of self-worth, self-respect, and self-honour and really know how to care for ourselves. Inner peace is a gift we give to ourselves. Another person cannot give it to us. If we always depend on other people to make us happy, we are at the mercy of that person's mood and depend on that person to give us a fix or an injection every time we need to feel good about ourselves. That is very wearing and leads to conflict and can often lead to relationship break ups.

The individual is responsible for how the self feels. If we can free ourselves from seeking approval this can lead to major life changing events. If we give ourselves the gift of self-worth and self-respect, then we can find the key to freedom from dependency on others. Only we ourselves alone have the power to set ourselves free by not seeking approval from others. Only we ourselves alone can empower our inner growth and self-esteem. Only we ourselves alone can make that first step to our own inner peace and happiness by letting the need for approval from others go.

Have an amazing day.

CHAPTER 3

Pressure cooker

Would you like to be free from raging anger?

Would you like to be free from conflicting situations?

Would you like to be free from defending yourself?

Would you like to be free from explaining yourself?

Would you like to be free from feeling guilty?

Would you like to be free from losing it when everyone else is at boiling point?

Our anger has been simmering for days and days. It has been burning slowly for what seems like an eternity. It has been building so intensely that we finally have to blow. The steam erupts from every part of our bodies and we lose control of ourselves. Our aim is to instantly scald the other person as they have scalded us – we will have to scald them.

The burning pressure that has been building up hour by hour, minute by minute, bubble by bubble, leaves us with no other option but to release our 'jiggy' valve loudly and uncontrollably. We let rip. We let go. We behave like a pressure cooker letting of stinging steam. We behave like a piston screaming manically from a steam engine. We behave like a fast, piercing whistle letting out a ferociously long whine.

A good while later, we cool down like someone has just poured chilly cold water over a pressure cooker. We begin to reflect and guiltily open the lid on what we did and what we said at the height of our anger. We ask ourselves what have we done? We ask ourselves what have we said? We ask ourselves what can we do to stop these outbursts and prevent our anger from ruining the relationships in our lives? We start to contemplate about how we can free ourselves from our anger.

We begin to learn that there are safety features that we can implement that won't scald ourselves and others too. We learn that there are easy instructions to follow that best suit our own inner pressure cooker. Simply things like taking plenty of time to exercise, to meditate, to socialise with true friends, to talk with someone who understands the real you, to do some gardening, to walk in nature, to have a nap, to go inside and listen to the inner voice within but most of all, do absolutely nothing but to stay still.

At a later time, we find that the anger begins to bubble up once again and we begin to simmer to boiling point. Don't worry. The safety valves will protect us. We know by now the best way to defuse a blow-out is to get ourselves out of that situation and avoid getting drawn into the argument. This is not easy to do as it takes time, patience and discipline. However, the main thing is to keep trying. We also know by keeping our energies balanced, we have more control over our emotions. This too takes hard work and real effort, but the rewards are bountiful. We really can find true inner peace in our lives by keeping a lid on our tempers.

The benefits of not releasing our pressure valve are life changing. We learn to remain in control. We learn to remain calm. We learn to remain grounded. Most of all, we learn to avoid the dreaded cooling down period which descends into defending ourselves, explaining ourselves and feeling guilty about an argument that could have been avoided. We gradually learn to keep our distance until the right time arises for any differences to be released at normal room temperature.

In short, by reflecting, meditating and going within, we can find answers to any conflict and we can turn any highly charged situation into one of calmness and love.

CHAPTER 4

You are worth it

Why not give yourself the gift of patience?

Valuing our self-worth and ourselves is so vital to our well-being that by opening ourselves to the treasures of the universe, we can change our lives and those of others. One treasure in the trove is patience. Why not give yourself the gift of beautiful patience? Learning patience can transform our lives. Learning patience can transform our inner selves. If we can learn to self-master our inner re-activeness to any kind of situation with gentle patience, we not only find peace on the inside but it helps to manifest peace on the outside.

Acquiring patience has an effect on every area of our lives, our relationships, our careers and most of all, acquiring patience teaches us to be patient with ourselves. When we learn patience, firstly with ourselves, we learn to look within and hear what our inner voice has to say to us, guiding us to follow our real true inner purpose, our real true inner instinct, our one true heart.

So how do we learn patience?

We slow down, we stop, and we learn to be still by meditating. We find time to make meditation part of our daily lives. By meditating, firstly we learn to be still, secondly we learn to be quiet, thirdly we learn to listen to our inner voice and finally, we learn the feeling of inner peace no matter what is happening around us. The inner feeling that we learn from meditating permeates into every minute of our day. The feeling becomes so strong that we will never want to feel any other way, or we never want to feel any negative thoughts permeate us.

We never want to feel any anger or frustration again. We learn to let everything go and learn to slowly go with the flow. We just let everything go with the tides of life. We learn not to react. We learn to live without anger. We learn to tune into the universe. We learn to patiently wait for things to settle down and turn itself around for our own good. The secret is to hang on no matter what the situation is or the outcome. We learn to hold the boat steady in the stormy waters of life until the waters of calmness are restored at the helm of inner balance.

How long does it take?

To achieve patience may take a whole lifetime but every outburst of impatience or anger can be soothed by healing that negative energy within us through mediation, reflection and the desire to change ourselves from within. We learn to take time out to reflect on our different outbursts for whatever reason. We learn to contemplate the triggers that set us off on the deep end – such as someone taking us for granted, someone trying to get inside our heads, or someone trying to bully us.

By learning patience within ourselves, we learn to distance ourselves from that person, from their words and from their deeds but showing and sending them love at all times. We learn to protect our inner balance from being corroded by negative language and people. Patience is the key. Patience teaches us not to control a situation. It teaches us not to force the outcome. The idea is that we set our boundaries and limits, that we know our core values and our self-worth, and that we protect them.

How do we do this?

We set out by protecting the inner self, by protecting our inner balance. Through the powers of meditation, we learn what it is like to be calm. Therefore, we learn what it is like to be patient. We learn to bring this feeling into every pore of our existence, into every ounce of our energy. This calmness that comes over us takes a lot of work, a lot of patience and persistence.

When we have accomplished this state of peace and serenity within us and learn to protect ourselves from any harmful imbalances, we can transform our lives into truly peaceful waters. We can tune into our real purpose in life. We learn to steer the wheel of our own ship. We learn to direct our own inner compass on our individual passage of life. The result is a total inner transformation occurs, a miracle occurs, and we find our Nirvana, our El Dorado, our Shangri-La.

CHAPTER 5

Ourselves vs others

The population of the western world is obsessed with comparing themselves with one another. We are obsessed with keeping up with our siblings, relations, neighbours, friends, colleagues whether it is materialistically, emotionally, academically even spiritually. We have to have in our house as much as they have or even more than they have. We have to have the last word in an argument because we know more than they do, and they don't understand us anyway.

If they are learning something new, then so will we. We think to ourselves who are they anyway doing an advanced course in Business, English or Spanish? Who do they think they are? Do they forget where they came from? Are they losing the run of themselves? Well, we will put them in their place. Well, we will take them down a peg or two.

This obsession with rivalry and keeping up with each other is in fact a heavy burden to carry and nobody wins. In fact, we alienate the person from our lives and we eventually fall out with them. The reason for this is that we are subconsciously preventing them from growing into the person that they want to be. We want to keep them in a box so we can feel better, so we can feel comfortable, so we can feel more secure because when everyone stays the same, we keep our power. When no one changes, we have control because no one is challenging our world, and no one is making us look at ourselves. The problem is we fear change.

But how about being bold and giving the people in our lives a break? Instead of being jealous and controlling, why not be encouraging and enthusiastic by wishing them well on their journey of self-discovery. Let them off, let them go. Don't feel afraid but feel excited that they want to go on an adventure which may change their whole lives, their whole outlook and their whole attitude to life. They might even give us the push to make changes in our own lives. Don't fear change, embrace it and think of it like this – it is better to be on the slow bus of change with everyone enjoying the journey together than waiting on a fast Mercedes car that may never turn up to drive us to some unknown destination alone, making us feel empty and unsatisfied.

Material wealth is not the answer. Acquiring money is not the answer. Yes, we need security and stability. But it is inner peace and growth that is the reason for us being in this life. Look at life as learning to deal with various people from all different backgrounds, experiences and values. Don't ever compare and don't ever be intimidated. Let us learn to be our authentic selves and accept ourselves as we really are.

But the secret is to get yourself into a zone where we would not like to be like anyone else no matter what they have, what they do or what they say. We need to learn to be comfortable in our own skin. We need to learn to be in satisfied in our own home. Let no one take away our feeling of uniqueness. Let no one take away our feeling of being special. This feeling makes up for all the materialistic, academic illusions that we sometimes look up to and value because we know and accept that deep inside ourselves we have our own individuality that no one anywhere in this whole universe can ever be like us.

Finally, we need to learn to shine our bright light of uniqueness everywhere and not lose ourselves in the darkness of the illusion of wealth that wraps itself around our identity and smothers us into the horrors of sameness and the mundaneness of being copycats. Let us brightly emit our splendid individuality and keep hold of it firmly because, then and only then, can we find our true path, our true way to inner peace and inner happiness.

CHAPTER 6

Finding happiness

Do you know the way to find contentment?
Do you know the way to find inner peace?

The first step is to ask ourselves a simple question, even though the question is an unusual one. But this question is so important to our well-being that we don't realise it. This question can change our whole life and lead us a place of inner calmness and inner well-being. What is that question?

The question is… How easy do we forgive ourselves and others?

We don't realise that by taking the huge step of forgiving ourselves and others, we show unconditional love to ourselves and those around us. Not forgiving others is a heavy burden to carry around with us day and night. Why not try to let it all go? Why not try to release the anger and the feeling of betrayal? Why not try to let go of all the negative experiences stored up in our memory from people and life? By doing this, we set ourselves free and give ourselves the permission to love ourselves and others. Now, it doesn't happen straight away, and the pain doesn't vanish overnight but by asking the question to forgive ourselves and others, we make the decision at least to think about it. This leads us then to the second step.

The second step is then to take the time out to reflect and forgive ourselves from all the hurt we caused others by putting it down to growth lessons and seeing these lessons as deepening our understanding of the self, people and life. We can often try to reflect on forgiving ourselves for the times we weren't there for others, for the times we didn't listen or show compassion to a friend, family or colleague. We can try to reflect on forgiving ourselves for not giving others the time and support they needed in tough times because we were wrapped up in our own worries, thoughts and needs. Reflection allows us time to heal the pain. Reflection allows us to forgive, forget and let go.

However, the reflection process opens up our old wounds and it may take a lot of time to learn to forgive and let it all go. This leads us to the next stage which is one of acceptance.

We learn to accept ourselves, who we really are and why we are really here. Through the process of forgiving ourselves and others, we learn tolerance, patience and understanding in our lives. We learn to rid ourselves of the guilt that we carry. We learn to be calm and let our inner peace envelop us. We learn to grow into fully complete, serene human beings. We learn to be courageous about the things we cannot change and about the things we can change. We learn truth. We learn integrity. We learn to just be and to be completely alive, feeling only inner stillness and inner peace. We learn our true identity.

By taking these steps, we are also on the way to changing and putting value on ourselves and putting value on our purpose in life. We learn that we have every right to be here and every right to have an opinion and have every right to have a say in what is happening in our own lives. But this is not an easy process. It takes time and a lot of belief and strength from within to let go of the baggage we carry. We have to try hard to believe that forgiveness will bloom in our garden of thought and will continue to bloom as time goes on. We will gradually learn to tend the budding flowers of love, care and kindness that grow within us. All of which stem from the seed of forgiveness.

Most of us recall the famous biblical words said on the cross: "Forgive them Father for they know not what they do." These lines are a great mantra to have in our heads when others are blind to our sensitivities, needs and feelings. If we can believe that there is so much going on in their heads that they cannot see beyond themselves, if we can learn to distinguish between what is other people's baggage and what is our own, we can then learn to differentiate between their pain and ours. If we can learn to wrap ourselves in a cloak of protection that only lets the positive in and keeps the negative out. Perhaps then we can all learn to forgive and forget, and eventually live in a state of inner peace.

It is up to us to protect ourselves from the thoughtlessness and bad deeds of others. It is up to us to put boundaries and limits around ourselves. It is up to us to say "no" that we do not accept others hurtfulness and painfulness. We also need to go that step further by forgiving them and letting all the pain and hurt go with love and light. It is up to us to get into the mindset that everything is for our highest good. We need to hang on in difficult moments, allow the situation to work itself out and also to allow it to turn around so that with time and space everyone can to see the best in every situation.

We need to let ourselves take a deep breath and count to ten. We need to believe there is a positive reason for everything. On the other hand, we need to believe that others have freedom of choice, the freedom to act as they wish. And hey, so do we. We just need to allow the time to elapse and let the situation slowly unfold. Most importantly, we need to protect ourselves from any backlash by remaining calm and still. Let time take its course and allow forgiveness to unfold slowly but surely in our lives.

Finally, by forgiving others, in time we let the bitterness go, we let the feelings of revenge go, we let the pain go. We eventually heal ourselves and turn our lives around. To heal the outside world, we need to heal the world inside first. Mediation is a great way to go within and reflect on our purpose, pains and plans for the future. Once we learn to forgive ourselves and others, we can de-clutter our pain and previous bad experiences from within, we will feel much lighter, happier and more in control of ourselves and our lives. So now is the time to forgive both ourselves and others, so let it all go. For we are all one.

CHAPTER 7

Expectation or stress

Expectations…

…internal…

…external…

…pressures…

…stress…

Do we have time to think of what actually stresses us out? Or is it just one long cycle of work, work, work and then a major overload in all areas of life, leading to a big explosion causing us to have a wobble, collapse and get ill. After a few days in bed (if we're lucky) most of us get better and then, off we go again on the vicious circle of stress, around and around and around we go. Others may not be so lucky.

What are we doing to ourselves? What is it all about? How do we get off the vicious roundabout of stress? What cost do these pressures have on our very own quality of life? Have we even got a balanced quality of life or are we letting society treat us like computers where societal so called 'norms' are downloaded in such a way that it dictates our internal and external expectations making us function like we are in some kind of matrix.

Let's look at all our expectations that we have upon our own shoulders from ourselves, others and society. Firstly, let's look at the internal expectations and pressures we have put upon ourselves; for example, pressure to be beautiful, slim, wear make-up, follow fashion trends, speak a certain way, have a certain job, have certain qualifications, have a big house, a new car, two holidays a year… Well, is it at all worth it when we have to work night and day to keep it all going? Let's ask ourselves whether we actually have a good quality of life or are our lives full of stress, pressure and torment?

Secondly, let's look at our external expectations from others and society? Pressure to keep up the facade of what others expect of us, the farcical facade of external perfection, to always be available, to never be able to say 'no', to always be polite, to always be happy, smiling, agreeable, and so on. Is society expecting us to be like a computer programme, daily downloading vast amounts of information in our minds, bombarding us with pictures, flooding our thoughts so much we can't think for ourselves. Are we becoming zombified? Are we becoming part of the cloud? Are we being dumbed down? Even computers have glitches, bugs and viruses. Let's just ask our society and others to give us a break. Let's ask society to let us think for ourselves and make our own decisions and live whatever way suits us. Let us ask society and others to allow us to make our own choices, take our own chances and make our own changes in our lives to be who we truly are.

Let us have our wobbles and outbursts in peace and allow us the time and space to see where we are going in life and for what reason we are going in a particular direction. Yes, space. Space is the magic word. We don't allow ourselves the space to think, to feel, and ask ourselves 'How actually am I today?' We do not give ourselves the space and time to reflect on the effect of these expectations and pressures society and others have on us. If we really took a close look, would we do what we do? If we really took the time to reflect on these internal and external pressures and asked ourselves to stop and get off the vicious circle of stress, wouldn't most of us jump off in a heartbeat?

But we don't stop. We just keep living by society's conditioning. The secret is to simplify our life, not complicate it. Let's just give ourselves the time and space to reflect on how important all these expectations are to us and reflect on how much is societal programming and conditioning, and how much is truly us. Let's make a choice, take a chance to change society's programme to one we chose ourselves.

How about bringing back time for ourselves and time for others? Bringing back community spirit where it's okay not to be okay, where it's okay to be open about pressures and trying to cope with all these expectations. Let people just be, let us just be people without all the trappings of society's baggage making us all overloaded and pressurised.

Eventually, this causes us to crash and forces the shut-down button because our firewall was just not able to keep up the facade any longer. As at the end of the day, we are not programmes. We are all powerful human beings with our own minds.

We don't need to be programmed. We should be free to make our own choices, live our lives in our own way and choose our own expectations. Simplification is the key. Go back to basics, to genuine relationships, to people being people without preloaded agendas expected by ourselves, others and society. We are all in this together. So, why are there mounting pressures, being pushed, pulled and moulded by these crazy expectations of material success and superficial pressures to think, act and be a certain way?

The system is overloading us time and time again. Now is the time to turn the societal system off, to stand back and reflect on the direction we're being pulled in and ask ourselves is this the direction we really want to go in and is this the way we want to live? We are not computers. We are not programmes. We are human beings with huge potential. But we allow our internal system to become overloaded over and over again. So now is the time to delete society and other people's files, to free ourselves by standing back and rebooting our own inner being, to follow our own inner purpose and not that of society and finally, waking up to who we truly are. We as people have the right to have our own freedom of choice, our own freedom to think, our own freedom to act and our own freedom to be ourselves in whatever way that may be.

Finally, let's reflect on one more thing. Are we really satisfied with the expectations and pressures we and society places on ourselves? Let's ask ourselves does it provide us with internal peace and calmness? Does it really fulfil our inner purpose, both individually and collectively?

Now is the time to reflect. Now is the time to act. Now is the time to be our own true selves, to jump off the treadmill of stress, pressure and tension. Above all else, now is the time to release our internal and external expectations, allowing us to be free of societal conditioning, programming and so-called 'norms'. Let us awaken to be our very own unique, individual beautiful self, live according to our own expectations and in our own individual, satisfying way.

CHAPTER 8

Listen

Do we listen to each other anymore?
Do we value the art of listening anymore?
Do we listen but cannot hear?

Do we listen to each other anymore, or are we just so full of noise in our heads about bills, children, jobs, relationships, sorting out the house, preparing meals, preparing for college, and meeting deadlines that we cannot hear what anyone is saying anymore? Is it that we listen to them, but we are unable to really hear and absorb anything anyone is saying to us despite our efforts?

What a big shame this is, as being listened to is a very special doorway that allows us to be understood, accepted and it enables us to share our inner thoughts, our inner feelings and our innermost turmoil about ourselves to others. If we are not listened to, over time there is a tendency to become frustrated and blocked as we have no release valve for what is going on in our heads or our hearts. This is because we have no one that listens to us, we have no one that values what we are saying. Maybe with a few tips we can learn to listen to each other again?

Four tips to help us listen to each other:

1) Firstly, we must learn to quieten the inner noise. We do this by learning to be quiet and still. We do this by emptying our heads and hearts of all external and internal noise during meditation, yoga, walking, even just sitting in a quiet place because if we don't learn to still the noise inside and learn to hear what others are saying, maybe we find that others find it hard to listen to us and hear what we are saying to them. Take some quiet time each day to relax and be alone. Start with ten minutes every day and after a while this time will become the most precious ten minutes of the day because you learn to listen to the inner beating of the heart and soul.
2) Secondly, when a friend/family member/partner is talking to us, let us ask ourselves the question: 'Am I really listening or am I just nodding my head with twenty other things going on in my head such as planning the day, thinking of texting someone, playing with my phone or thinking what to do at the weekend?' Let us take a moment to stop and think, to observe what is going on in our heads when someone is telling us something important about a relationship issue, work problems or are in need of advice. Let us stop the noise in our heads and give them a kind ear by listening to every word in detail, as we never know when it is our turn for

someone to listen to us about our issues, dilemmas and problems.

3) Thirdly, place value on those friends who listen to us in our time of difficulty. We all have our faults but for those friends who pick up the phone at any time day or night and just listen to us, letting us pour out our troubles – these friends are worth their weight in gold as listening seems to be a dying art in the days of many distractions from social media to texting to Viber to WhatsApp. Every conversation or message has to be quicker, shorter, to the point that no one seems to have any time to listen to what anyone else has to say. So, let us try and take time out in the week to meet and have a good conversation with the special people in our lives and maybe learn to appreciate and value their gift of listening to us and for us to really, really listen to them.

4) Finally, look out for friends, a family member, or a partner, especially when there is a party, birthday, wedding or Christmas. If in company at a party, look for signs that someone may need closer attention or may need someone to listen to them. Sometimes we can be so alone in a group. Sometimes we can be surrounded by everyone, but no one sees us, no one sees our pain. We may be feeling invisible. This is not a nice place to be in. But when we feel alone, sometimes we don't recognise it ourselves

> until someone asks us 'Are you okay?' and then we blurt it all out and from them we receive the gift of being listened to.

We are so relieved to actually have found someone who has taken the time to really listen to us. We may find ourselves crying, we may even find ourselves laughing at the end of the conversation but from one empathetic question, we may get whatever it was off our chest and as a result we feel refreshed, renewed and we feel ready to restart our journey all over again maybe even enjoy the party. As a result, this can start a chain reaction where we then learn to reciprocate and look out for other friends who need a friendly ear and someone just to listen to them.

CHAPTER 9

Our True Purpose

Why we should let go and live our dreams?

Every single one of us is born with a purpose. We may be well into our forties and fifties before we even realise what we are really meant to be doing for the rest of our lives. Everything we did up to now is preparation for this time. It is now time to take up our real purpose in life. We have served our apprenticeship. Now it is time to master life and understand why we are here at all. Life is really only beginning.

Some people go back to education and retrain in something they always wanted to do but couldn't due to life's demands so now have a second chance in their forties to start again. We may go back to college to retrain in anything from midwifery to teaching to being a special needs assistant, to setting up our own business. It can range across many different areas. But it is in doing this, we tune into our life's true purpose that genuinely sets us free to be who we really want to be.

Once we are doing our purpose, we are in our zone of truth. We are alive and life really becomes easier to handle. We are in the universal flow and in touch with our true essence. We are being our true selves because we are doing what we came here to do. Doors open that were impossible to open before now. The right people come into our lives. Events in our lives just fall into place effortlessly. We begin to understand and to learn what life is really all about. We have learned to be truly grateful as we know how difficult things can be when we were doing our so-called apprenticeship of life.

Now we have a chance to become masters of ourselves and situations. We have a chance to become the person who we were always meant to be. Now we have a chance to awaken and become a living force to be reckoned with. We have a chance to arrive at the pinnacle of our true state of being.

Once we have made the decision to pursue our purpose, we can now trust that whatever happens is meant to happen and if we understand that life is all about acquiring lessons. We understand that things which may go wrong, are only to make way for the better things to come. We understand that the negative energy is being cleared to make way for the positive energy to manifest itself. Hence, we learn to trust and release to the outcome. We surrender to life's path and all its miraculous events. We become one with the beating heart of life's mission. We become one with ourselves and all eternity.

Follow that dream.

Don't ever stop no matter what happens for that is our true purpose calling us. Keep dreaming. Let us allow ourselves to dream regularly, to imagine how much easier life would be if we were doing our dream job or being in a dream relationship with our true love and having all the right people around us. It can be done. It is within our reach.

We just need to trust and let go. We need to trust in the universal flow of life that situations will happen once we put it out there. So now is the time to take action and put in place the necessary actions to let life take its true course as it was always meant to happen and finally be who we are really meant to be. We must finally awaken to our true purpose and live our dream life.

CHAPTER 10

Dreams can come true

We all dream of the life we would love to have with more money, bigger houses, faster cars, more holidays abroad. We all think some days that if we had a magic wand, we would know exactly what we would conjure up. We would know in a flash all the things we'd love to have. But do we realise that the universe is like a magic wand and if we visualise daily the things we need and actively picture our lives the way we want them, we can manifest our dreams into reality because what we think about, we attract. A lot of us may be familiar with the book called 'The Law of Attraction' written by Rhonda Byrne, a self-help book on the effects of thinking positively. In short, she wrote that positive thoughts attract positive results.

We are aware that thinking positively can sometimes be difficult but it's a really great habit to get into. If we can possibly eliminate all negative thoughts about ourselves and others and fill our minds with great positivity about the lives we truly deserve, including the kind of people we want in our lives, then we can make it happen by casting the spell of manifestation and sticking to our dreams no matter what happens.

Yes, it is hard. Yes, it takes time. Manifestation takes work. Nothing happens overnight. Some people may find it easier to make a picture board by filling it with photos or images of what and who they want to have in their lives. By looking at our picture board and thinking positively a few times a day, we can cast a manifestation spell and eventually the universe transforms our dreams into a new sparkling reality. Well, is it that easy?

We usually start off positively but like everything else, it takes a lot of persistence, patience and practice. The trick is not to stop believing it will happen. We may actually feel that our lives are getting worse rather than better. The universe puts challenges in our way, like difficulties with our friends, the ending of a long-term relationship, divorce, financial difficulties but this is the universe clearing out our treasure trove of woes to manifest for us a wonderful new life.

It is very important to hang on and ride the magic carpet of life as the universe works very slowly but it does work, and it eventually attracts the life we'd like to lead and the people we'd like to have in our lives. The secret is to never give up trying to manifest the life we want. It takes great strength to make our dreams come true but one thing to remember is that if we dream of meeting the right partner, finding the best job we ever had, having all the money we need, we have to absolutely one hundred percent believe that it will really happen.

We must have total faith in the universe's power to manifest our very own dreams. One thing to remember is that people have free will and we cannot interfere with that.

What seems to work for a lot of people is that instead of asking for specifics – such as asking for someone tall, dark and handsome with loads of money – instead, a better way is to ask the universe to bring us great love, great abundance, great peace, great harmony and great happiness, etc.

Vagueness seems to work best when casting the manifesting spell to conjure up our new magic filled life. But we need to have total trust in the universe as like attracts like. Positive attracts positive and vice-verse. Thinking positively takes a lot of discipline and self-control. We all know that some days this can be difficult to do but when negative thoughts dominate our minds, we have to learn to switch the channel and eliminate the onslaught of negative thinking. Some people use prayers, some people use affirmations like saying, 'I am safe and secure at all times', 'I am loved and I am love', 'I have a right to have an easy life' – use whatever affirmation works for you.

The message here is to be aware of our thought process. Negative thinking is a bad habit, but we can change these patterns by finding our own switch to turn off the big black cauldron of bad thoughts bubbling in our minds and remember positive attracts positive. So just let the magic happen. Let us wave the universe's magic wand without fear and let miracles happen. Remember, it takes time. Be patient.

One other thing to remember is that we cannot manifest a perfect life for others. We cannot interfere with others' free choice. We are only able to attract what we desire rather than what others desire. However, remember and trust that we can make our very own wildest dreams come true. We can, believe it or not, change our lives because by changing our thoughts on the inside, we can change the world we live in on the outside.

Happy dreaming!

CHAPTER 11

Satisfaction

We are a consumer society, we buy, buy, buy from food to furniture to fashion but are we ever satisfied? Are we filling a gap that is deep inside that we don't address? Do we just keep plugging the gap with material goods? This is like a quick fix to far more complicated issues. We are superficially putting a plaster on our wounds and not really using any ointment to heal the infection.

We need to look deeper within as to what is really going on because if we don't, we become addicted to quick fixes and all we're doing is fixing our habit and not healing the addiction. As people, we all have our addictions and this huge need in us for satisfaction with external hits is avoiding the real issue.

Do we go through the day going from one addiction to another, drinking coffee, eating chocolate, have a glass of wine or two, buying some new clothes to get a lift? Always looking for a life, looking to satisfy the craving of our needs. If we keep expecting external hits to satisfy us, we will always feel frustrated and needy. Our lives will be driven by the need to earn money to satisfy our habit. Our lives will be driven by the need to always change, update and seek the answer from the outside world when all we have to do is look within.

The same addiction can be applied to people because our addiction needs approval from others. We need an external fix of approval but again, that only temporarily soothes the wound until we are once again needing a hit. We never really get satisfied, and it becomes a vicious circle. We are trapped in an addictive cycle that imprisons us in a certain way of life – a life of need, need, need.

Wouldn't you love to be free of over-dependence on temporary satisfaction and quick fixes? All answers to our problems are found within. All solutions are inside of us. Our addictions can be cured. We can learn to be free. How does it work? We must learn to listen to our inner voice by doing some reiki, yoga, meditation classes, long walks on the beach – really learn to slow down and re-prioritise our lives as to what and who is really important in our lives. Life can then change for the better. Our needs will change, our world will change and the way we think, and view life will change. We become far less needy as a person, more able to manage our finances, and we become less demanding on ourselves and others. We learn detachment. We go with the universal flow of life so that we learn to feel safe and secure at all times – no matter what is happening around us. We no longer will have the need to fill our emotional, mental, and physical insecurities. We no longer crave the reassurance, approval, need to be humoured or to humour other people to get what we need. We become a whole, complete, functioning human being. We learn to be free. We learn inner satisfaction and we learn inner peace. We learn to live in moderation. We learn to live and remain in balance. By changing the pattern of our thoughts, by going within, we change the pattern of our behaviour and actions. We change our own lives. We no longer feel the need to serve our neediness. We find true satisfaction that flows in abundance through our veins enriching or lives and others lives. We come home to our true selves.

CHAPTER 12

Love ourselves

How do we learn self-respect?
How do we learn self-worth in relationships?

The secret to loving ourselves in a healthy way is to firstly learn to say no to others without feeling guilty; secondly, put boundaries around ourselves to protect our energies; thirdly, control our negative thoughts about others and ourselves and to always keep them positive. These steps are not easy to achieve. These steps are not easy to keep balanced. It takes a lot of effort to keep our energies balanced and keep in control of ourselves and also protect ourselves from other people's baggage.

This is a juggling game of ups and downs, but the secret is to persist and be sure to get plenty of space and rest. Today's lifestyle is so busy we get little time to reflect on how we feel about the effects of others' behaviour on our inner selves. Reflection takes time and can be painful but well worth it. When we reflect on others' reactions, we learn to gather strength again to say no, we learn to gather the strength again to reinforce our boundaries, we learn to transmute our negative thoughts by changing the channel and letting all negativity go, replacing them with positive vibrant thoughts and feelings. By having a rest, we learn to wipe the slate clean and start again.

By using judgement or discernment to make a decision about something or someone in your life, try not to make a negative judgement such as putting the other person down. We need to learn to try and detach any negative actions and negative thoughts from the person and let go with love and peace. In a perfect world this is not hard to do but in everyday life, to live detached from the effects of people's behaviours is very difficult to do and it takes a lot of time and practice.

We have to decide if a person's actions are good for us while trying not to judge the person or think negatively about them. By doing this we learn how to deal with people and interact with them in a tolerant way. We try to get to know them before letting them in, before we get to know them intimately or have a relationship with them. We learn to protect ourselves. We learn to take our time getting to know people. We learn to take our time letting them in using discernment, intelligence, knowledge from meeting other people that we've met before. We try to be sensible, especially when meeting potential partners, trying to be shrewd, astute, and careful by assessing people's actions and their effect on us.

Traits to look out for are things such as if they are controlling then they will always be controlling, if they don't seek to be a better person by choosing an honourable path they will not change. People need to want to change, want to be better, want to listen, want to take the path of temperance and moderation, want to take a higher path, want to fight their demons and take the long route and not a quick fix. The honourable life is a long journey, but a worth-while journey and we have to be confident enough to let others go if their road doesn't change for the better so as to leave space for new people and new lessons.

Before we commit to a relationship, we should take a lot of time before we really know the person. We need to be discerning. This is also extremely hard to do as most of us rush in headfirst. Relationships are not easy and can be massive learning curves and even bigger lessons. But a lot of couples say, and maybe it's true, that we just know when we meet the right person and all plans to be discerning go out the window. Maybe the safest way to act is to protect ourselves as best we can. One thing that is very important is to remain financially independent. This is crucial and could solve a lot of arguments.

Financial matters are where the problems start. If it is at all possible, remaining financially independent of one another is the jewel in the crown of any relationship. By all means, sharing the bills and costs should go without saying but for both people in the relationship. For both parties' sake, in theory having a safety fund is vital and reassuring should difficulties occur. However, in practice it can be hard to have any spare cash to save.

Emotional independence is hard to achieve in any loving relationship because when we give someone our heart, we are very much likely to emotionally co-depend on each other. This can be scary for a lot of people and leaves us open to all types of pain such as fear of rejection, fear of not being good enough to be loved, losing confidence that no one else would find us attractive, fear of being alone. But love in a relationship brings all these issues up and as couples, we must learn to heal the emotional pain. This can be a result of pain from previous lifetimes as well as this one.

We need to learn to heal our emotional pain and learn to love ourselves in a healthy way first before we can really love and emotionally connect with another person. Bear in mind that love in any relationship is as much about pain as it is as much about love because there are times when we are not happy with them and not happy without them. What does all this mean and how is it all worth it?

We need to understand ourselves and our limits. We need to know our boundaries, our values, our temperament, our weaknesses, our limits. But love finds a way. It cannot be said often enough but it will only continue to grow if the love is not tainted with mistrust, unfaithfulness, selfishness, physical, emotional or mental abuse. For love to grow it needs understanding, commitment, hard work and belief in each other. When the relationship becomes abusive and destructive, it sours and destroys each-others love. It is necessary to always have the fundamental belief that hurting our partners is the last thing that we would ever want to do and doing everything possible to protect each other from the downward spiral of destructive love.

It seems very complicated but if our limits are being tested over and over again, how can we protect ourselves? Most of us stay too long for one reason or another in our relationships as the fear of being alone is much greater and takes a lot of strength, especially when there are children involved. But society's relationships are changing, and we see multi-parents in a family relationship.

As society is more complex than before, children are more likely to have a stepfather and/or stepmother due to divorce being an option previous generations did not have. But even with divorce being an option, love is still something we all strive to have. To love our other half and share a life together is still very much possible when the love remains positive and constructive and is what both partners should always try to achieve in their relationship.

Love is not a mathematical equation; it is very much a language of its own. It is based on both parties mutually needing the same thing. This is also why getting to know one another is so important to any relationship having a chance. But once we fall, it is very hard to keep all these limits to protect ourselves but as they say – we know many reasons to leave but we only need one reason to make us stay.

Many believe when you really love someone you will as Sting from the Police states, 'when you love someone set them free' and also try not to be a slave to love and that person because then it moves into dependency and destruction. That is why we all need to keep the relationship healthy and independent.

Yes, there are ups and downs but if we hold the belief that we are protected by a greater power than us and that we are safe no matter what happens, then we can survive the break-up of any relationship. Yes, people and partners let each other down but knowing that we can get up and face life again is the essence of self-love, self-trust and having self-worth. Self-sufficiency is vital and needs to be a priority too.

If we hold the belief and understand that no one can destroy us – unless we allow them – we can build the life we want, live the way we were meant to live because people should enhance your life, bring positive energy, laughter, love and happiness and not the opposite. A constructive, transforming kind of love is the opposite because it changes lives, changes people, changes the world…

Trust.

CHAPTER 13

Ways to cope

Impatience triggers stress and stress triggers impatience.

Did you know that triggers of impatience lead to the triggers of stress and vice versa? The more stressed we are, the more impatient we are and the more impatient we are, the more stressed we are. The two go hand in glove. If we learn to control our impatience, we can learn to control our stress levels. If we learn to control our stress levels, we can learn to control our impatience. The question is whether there is a cure for stress. Is there a secret to feeling calm, relaxed, and chilled in all areas of our lives?

Impatience and stress trigger emotional outbursts.

Do you find yourself screaming down the phone at some call centre representative who may just scream back at you and both of you find that in the end you are getting nowhere fast? Do you find yourself getting impatient and stressed with the waiter or waitress in a restaurant because you are so tired, hungry or hungover? Do you find yourself getting agitated and irritable with the bank official who, by the way, is not responsible for the queues in the bank or the bank bailout? Well, these emotional outbursts get us nowhere. They just launch a thousand missiles into our bunker of impatience and blow our stress levels into oblivion. What can we do, we ask ourselves as we did not ask for these problems either?

We may not be able to control the ills of society but one thing we can definitely do is to control our emotional outbursts by learning to understand our impatience and learning to understand what actually stresses us out. How can we do that?

Impatience and stress trigger procrastination.

We all put things on the long finger but more so when we are stressed because we are already overloaded and anything extra to be done is always put off until the never, never because the body, mind and soul need recovery time until they can start something new. If and when we find ourselves procrastinating when we need to study, prepare a presentation or have a deadline, we should ask ourselves – Am I already overloaded? What can we do?

Impatience and stress trigger the ego.

When we are impatient and stressed, the ego raises its dark head. The ego is our remote control and with this we like to press other people's buttons to show them who is in charge. We can get sarcastic, we can put conditions on people, we can try and control all outcomes to satisfy our needs to be the winner and the absolute best. We are the overall ruler and everyone else are just slaves to our needs. This does not sound good and we deny that this is who we really are. How can we change ourselves?

Impatience and stress trigger ill health.

Impatience tells us and can be looked upon as a barometer for our stress levels. As we all know, stress is a killer and the long terms effects of stress can lead to anxiety, depression and a possible break down. What can we do?

The secret is to take time out and learn who we really are on the inside and learn to be our authentic self. If we give ourselves enough time to go within and discover our inner voice by meditating and teaching ourselves calmness, we can learn inner peace. There are many, many ways to relax and learn inner stillness. All we need to do is to introduce one or two ways slowly into our lives and the let the magic happen. Enjoy the journey back to your real peaceful inner self.

CHAPTER 14

Measuring success

The world seems obsessed with measurement to the point that even the wine glass has an exact measurement drawn on the glass just in case we get an extra drop too much. What is it all about?

There seems to be an obsession with external standards such as food hygiene, the environment, safety at work, etc. It is all about regulation this, regulation that and keeping high standards. This is all great and all for our own good as it makes our lives run more efficiently, keeps us safe from food poisoning and keeps us from any unnecessary injuries at work and so on. That is a good thing, right?

Well, what about our internal standards, values, moral code, principals? How do we measure them? How do we measure kindness, love, wisdom, integrity?

In its race for wealth and materialistic goods, has the world forgotten the existence of internal values like inner beauty, inner truth and our inner light? Unfortunately, the world measures success externally. No longer do we value loyalty and the ability to share and care for each other. We teach our children in school to be competitive and individualistic. We teach them the attitude to think of themselves only and to ask, 'What is in it for me?' We teach them economic and monetary values of wealth and of materialistic measurement.

We teach them to compete against each other. Well ok, competition is healthy if it helps students to reach their maximum potential but not if it teaches students to judge each other by putting someone down for not being in the top five percent in the country or comparing their results to their friends who have different abilities and strengths to themselves. Everybody's abilities are as individual as our fingerprints. No two people have the same ability in everything they do. Thus, to judge and compare students or people on not having this and that ability is a negative trait in schools in particular and in society in general.

We need to go back to measuring our internal values and placing a value on them. As a society, we have lost our way. We have forgotten to be human and cherish internal principals, internal morals, internal values and internal standards. We need to go within and do a deep search to find them again. This takes a lot of work and a lot of time.

We also need to slow down and look at why we do the things we do and ask ourselves is it worth working long hours just for wealth and materialistic things when we have no quality of life, when we don't see our families, when we don't get to enjoy a walk on the beach or take time out with a friend because we are too busy paying for all our external possessions.

External wealth cannot buy happiness or love as happiness and love belong to the internal values of life. Until we can forgo our addiction to external possessions, go within and search for the inner light, the world will remain the same. Why does society pass judgement and put people without wealth, without materialistic goods on the last rung of the ladder of popularity?

Society needs to reflect, change its mind-set by cleaning up its act and ridding itself of greed and corruption, by going within and reflecting on whether we are being who we really are or do we put on a big act to humour the people around us and to fit in. No wonder we explode with frustration and anger as it takes a lot of energy to be fake and false and put on an act. Let's make a small change and let's ask ourselves who we really are. Are we honestly happy with ourselves and the way we act with people? If we answer 'no', let us learn to be true to ourselves and let us learn to be false to no one. Let us learn to value our inner wealth as it provides us with boundaries that protect us from losing our own uniqueness, identity and maintaining who we really are.

CHAPTER 15

Your other half

Do you know your twin flame?

Do you know how to attract in your twin flame?

Do you know that now is the time of the twin flame reunions?

Everyone has another half, another being that completes them otherwise known as their twin flame. A twin flame is different to a soul mate as we can have many soul mates, but we can only have one true twin flame. The difference between the love from our twin flame's heart and the love from someone's ego are complete opposites. Love from the ego is destructive and love from the heart is constructive. Love from the heart is unconditional and the ties of this love can never be broken. Did you know that twin flames were once one entity many moons ago and are now reuniting all over the world?

True love from the heart of twin flames has nothing to do with their looks, their money, their job, their friends. It has all to do with the connection they both feel when they are together. No one else fully completes them like that person. No one else looks at them like that person. No one else sees them like that person.

Now more than any other time in history, twin flames are coming together to show the rest of the world about valuing unconditional love from the heart rather that valuing romantic love from the ego. Therefore, people who are single, divorced, or separated, please don't give up hope as now is the perfect time to attract your one and only true twin flame. Simply start by opening up the heart chakra, believing in him or her and by sending out positive signals to the universe. In doing this, we get positive signals back. However, we do need to prepare ourselves for the arrival of our twin flame.

Firstly, we need to be able to feel love in our hearts for love to find us. Secondly, we need to love ourselves first before someone else can love us. If we don't love ourselves, it can block us from attracting our twin flame's love. Thirdly, we need to think of our twin flame often and send them love from our hearts – even if we haven't met them yet.

The universe will then connect the twin flames, and both can share the love vibe subconsciously. The love vibe will attract them into our lives. Coincidental meetings will start happening to bring both flames together. And the rest can be left up to the universe.

Now the question is – what happens when we meet our twin flames? Is it happy ever after? The answer of course is no. The course of true love never runs smoothly. The course of the twin flame love is filled with obstacles and upheavals. There are several different stages to the reunion once they recognise each other. The first three stages are the most difficult.

The stages are:

1) testing stage
2) crisis stage
3) runner dynamic stage
4) surrender stage
5) radiance stage
6) harmonizing stage

The purpose of the first stage, called the testing stage, is to clear conflict about outdated beliefs in how relationships are supposed to be. True love has no conditions, no restraints. There is no right and wrong there just is.

The second stage is the crisis stage which deals with conflict between the ego and the heart. The ego finds it hard to accept a higher expression of love and doesn't want to embrace the higher love of their twin flame. Fear and stubbornness lead to anxiety and triggers regular dysfunctional emotional patterns between the twin flames. But throughout this cycle they come together to make up, make amends and reunite.

At the third stage, called the runner dynamic stage, the relationship is again victimised by the ego. The runner twin withdraws and blocks out the other twin. This withdrawal can mean the twin flames may never reach the next three stages unless the outcome of the universe is to reconnect them.

To get to the fourth stage, the surrender stage, both flames have to believe and trust that the union will happen in its own time. However, the runner twin is given time, space and freedom to grow at his or her own pace. The surrendered twin still holds a torch for him/her but is also free to fully explore life.

At stage five (the radiance stage), the ego dies, and the force of pure love takes over. The twins once romantic love awakens into divine love.

Finally, at the sixth and last stage, the harmonizing stage, both twins merge into unconditional love and create a third energy that guides others to open their hearts to search for their own twin flame and learn to believe in the freedom of unconditional love.

CHAPTER 16

Have it all

Say to yourself:

I have a right to be here.
I have the right to be happy.
I have my own uniqueness to offer.
I am a special person.
I have a value that is priceless.
I am equal to everyone else.
I can have it all.

Good self-esteem means that we know our worth and value ourselves. Low self-esteem means we don't know our own worth. What happens if we change these negative assumptions to positive affirmations, if we switch from negative thoughts to positive thoughts? We can change our lives.

The law of attraction really works. Our thoughts have a positive charge and the universe picks this charge up. Sending out a positive charge means receiving a positive outcome. Sending a negative charge means receiving a negative outcome. It is that simple.

By breaking the negative opinions of ourselves, we can change how we think about ourselves, we can change how we feel about ourselves and we can change how we react to others. Instead of being full of anxiety and overloaded with negativity, we can learn to control it by filling our thoughts with only positive thoughts, ideas and opinions. Instead of releasing a whole load of negative emotions and frustrations, we stay in the moment, acknowledging that we feel anxious, but we release it to the universe and change our thought patterns to only positive ones. We don't allow our thoughts to control us. We control our thoughts. We switch the channel.

If we can think positively, feel positive, act positively and get positive reassurance from our family, peers and friends, we can change how we feel about ourselves. It is all based on our own belief, trust, and confidence in our inner abilities to achieve our goals. It is our ability to keep trying and never giving up on our dreams and visions for a better life. We have the right to have a good quality life. We have the right to have an easy life. We have the right to feel good about ourselves on the good days as well as on the bad days. By balancing our thoughts and by raising our self-esteem, we can change the lows into a balanced healthy feeling about ourselves. Our own balanced self-esteem is all about loving ourselves, being comfortable with ourselves and being true to ourselves any time, any place or anywhere. Learning to flow with the river of life to find the shore of our true nature.

Why do we have an obsession to control, push and pull situations to achieve a fixed outcome? Whereas if we just let it all go, relaxed and released situations to reach their naturally outcome in a natural flow everything would work out much, much better. We would all react in a softer way and everyone would feel one billion percent calmer in the end. But what are we like? We tense up, we get irritated and we go against all the advice in the world to relax and refuse absolutely point blank to release our drowning man's grip of control to an external force like the universe.

Instead, with every ounce of strength we try to own every beating impulse, every brilliant idea, every bouncing action. Then we try to imprison every single thing to the chains of control – as everything we have belongs to us and we always know what's best in every situation… We always, always try to control the outcome because we know what's best as it's all me, me, me. Our rigid attitude is that no one owns my stuff, my idea, my house, my car, my everything, my life. No one knows better than me. Is this the way we actually are? Do we actually know what is better for us or is there a better way?

Well, that may be a slight exaggeration, but you can see where I am coming from. However, the powers that be believe that if we relaxed more and went with the flow of the universe, released our urge to control situations and outcomes, and behaved less stressful in situations, we would be more relaxed. In turn, these things would have less impact on us, and we would have less negativity in our lives. A prime example is when we are getting an injection from the nurse. In the surgery when getting an injection, the nurse always asks us to relax before the injection punctures our skin because if we are relaxed rather than all tensed up the injection is not as painful as the muscles are more relaxed.

The same idea applies when trying to control outcomes and situations because if we relaxed and took a chill pill, not only do we ourselves come into our own truly relaxed state but so does everyone else around us. Don't we all work better when we are feeling in the flow, smiling, talking slowly, breathing easily and taking our time? We can all reap boundless benefits by releasing all cares and worries to the universe and resisting all attempts to control situations and outcomes. Once we have done all we can, is it not up to the powers that be?

Anyway, they say that life falls into place much more easily when we are in our true natural flow. So why not let us try and trust our very own true inner nature to bring us all to the best possible outcome because when we let all outcomes reach their own final resting place, the best situation for everyone occurs. Many believe that the only thing that needs to be controlled is money. Everything else has a natural flow, just like water twisting and turning its way along the bed of soil and rock on its journey until it eventually finds its true path to the sea – its natural destination.

The same applies to our own lives as we twist and turn around the obstacles of life. We must forge our way through. As we try to work our way around the obstacles in a slow persistent flowing kind of movement, the outcome actually reaches its own true full potential. As you know water is a simple compound made up of H_2O, unlike the complex nature of say K[Pt(NH3)Cl5] potassium ammine penta chloroplatinate, water is made up of only two elements, hydrogen and oxygen yet it wears down the hardest rock and is vital and essential to life on this planet. Water just ebbs and flows. It moves around obstacles, wearing and eroding everything in its flow – fluidity finding its true path and existing in its own true essence on its way to join the sea.

We can do exactly the same. We can find the way back to our own true nature as we flow in the sea of life by gently preparing, plotting, planning our individual course, navigating our very own voyage. Allowing the sea of life to bring us safely back to the shores of our true nature that knows no control, only fluidity forever forward moving, flowing and following our own true life's path and purpose, because that's the only real journey we really know and desire.

The path and course of our life's plan should always flow without any force, control or resistance – just moving forward with fluidity and natural flow. Is it not time to go back to our true nature and natural flow of living? We can do so by finding and following our very own true purpose, by releasing all our control over all final outcomes and situations. After all we can only do our best and the rest, as they say, is up to the powerful all-knowing universe.

CHAPTER 17

Understanding life

Well, one thing we all know for sure about life is that we all know it is very short. Some days we may be glad that it's short! One thing that may help us on those kinds of days is remembering that we are all here for a purpose. Also, we are all here to learn who we truly are because we have forgotten our true connection to the universe and the source of all being. At birth we undergo a certain kind of amnesia which deletes all memory of our past experiences here on earth and all experiences of our past lives become completely forgotten.

Many of us are old souls who have been here many times. Sometimes in dreams we can get images of our past lives, but it can be hard to make sense of what has happened once we wake up. We may find ourselves even asking why we are here. As you may have guessed, there are many answers to this question but some of us believe that we are all here for one main purpose – that is to help ourselves and the planet earth, also called Gaia (mother nature), return back to her and our true spiritual nature. But the majority of us have lost our way on the path of spirituality.

At the moment at this special time in history, many of the old ancient tribes of American Indians, African tribes, Aborigines have foretold the coming of this time called the Ascension Process. In this, we will all evolve once again and take up our higher purpose to help ourselves, others and the planet return to our God spark and to its rightful place in the divine universe.

As above, here is another simple way to understand the ascension process. It may also be called the awakening. We awaken to our true purpose and our true calling. Within the midst of our awakening, the cloud of clarity starts to lift. We have many moments when we are gifted with the grace of understanding that this process, which may last over our lifetime, is happening to us and others so we need to hang on when the cloud descends again, and our sight becomes foggy again. It is no easy ride through the many twists and turns of life's lessons, but we need to remember that we are all in this together for our own higher purpose and for the higher purpose of the planet.

That's all well and good, but how does that pay the bills and sort out our emotional and mental wellbeing, as well as the financial problems? How does knowing this and undergoing this process help us through the daily grind of life? Well, many of the great prophets of the past including Buddha, believed that we have chosen our lives, we have chosen our lessons, we have chosen to be here to evolve and ascend at this amazing time in history. We have chosen to evolve for a higher purpose. So, if we understand life's purpose from this perspective, it may help us understand why we are here.

How do I know I am awakening?

One way to find out is to tune into the divine energies all around us by going within and learning to listen to our inner self. We need to learn how to connect to the source by finding some quiet time to drown out the hum-drum noise that surrounds us every day. Time out is essential. It is not only good for our body and mind, but it is also good for our soul.

If ignored, the soul cries out to be heard, to help us through our ups and downs in life. We are the captain of our ship. This stirs our head, stirs our heart but most of all, stirs and guides our beautiful soul to connect without consciousness to our higher self and to the source of all being.

Another way to guide us through our stair of ascension is to trust that no matter what happens, we are on our journey, on our way to the destination of finding out about the most wonderful emotion ever experienced, which is a four-letter word – love. It may sound simple but as we know when we reflect that love is anything but simple. That is what we are all here to learn. The greatest love story ever told is the one about humanity finding her true course, her true destination back to the light. We are here to learn to love ourselves, love each other. Whatever difficulty we find ourselves in is only a mirror reflecting a block of blocked energy back at us, a reminder for us to take time to reflect and heal ourselves to remember who we truly are.

If we hold the belief that there is no failure, there is no doubt or fear, only blocks preventing us from loving ourselves and others. These blocks can be healed through meditation, yoga, and reiki. There are many different ways to heal our inner self. We just have to find the one that suits us best and keep doing it. But on a dark day remember that there is a higher purpose which we chose to be part of at this time. We have chosen our family, we have chosen our lives, we have chosen our path in life and we are responsible for the quality of our lives.

Follow your inner voice and learn to love yourself and others unconditionally for everything we experience is the sum of our thoughts, transferred into feelings and manifested into actions which will beyond doubt, be mirrored back to us. Remember not to hurt anyone and let love flow within us like a bouncing, bubbling, breath-taking stream of water flowing majestically down the mountain stream of life, flowing to its one true purpose – to ascend to the higher oceans of humanity to be once again one with the universe at the source of all being.

CHAPTER 18

Transform, revive and refresh

The only way to transform ourselves, our lives, our relationships is by accepting, understanding and loving ourselves unconditionally. We can then set ourselves free once and for all by truly loving ourselves and being one with ourselves. Only then can we experience healing loving relationships in our lives. Relationships fall apart when we look to others to fill the gap and heal the pain in our soul and heart. But is that not the way it has always been done?

The problem is that looking to someone else to sort out our insecurities and fears, is the start of our emotional downward spiral that twists painfully out of control into negative emotions like pain, anger and jealousy. An example is if we need our partner to protect us from our fears, it may eventually drive him or her away. The relationship becomes a prison of negativity and eventually leads to separation because the loving energy is smothered, stifled and cannot grow, so it dies. Other people cannot heal our pain – only we can do that.

How do we set ourselves free?

The secret to loving ourselves is by accepting ourselves wholly and completely, avoiding self-judgement and self-criticising, learning to trust ourselves, by understanding that every experience is for our highest good and that every event in our life is a lesson and will deepen our understanding of ourselves and others. The secret is to go within and reflect on who we are, why we do the things we do, if we don't like the things we do we should ask for help and seek out ways to complete our inner authentic self. We need to give ourselves time to think, reflect and contemplate on our inner well-being. Then we can change ourselves, our relationships and our lives for the better.

Why do we have this pain?

The reason for the pain we carry is not only from our life's experience but because we carry negativity from our past lives as well as from this one. We were once one with the source of all there is and many millions of years ago, our soul separated from this paradise and started a journey of evolution. Our soul carries the pain of that separation and this pain arises in our loving relationships with other people especially in our relationship with our immediate partners. The secret is to allow ourselves and others time and space to heal the pain even if it means separating from each other for a while. We need to heal ourselves from within first before we can begin to know, attract and experience a healing constructive love in our lives.

What do we need to do?

Such as when a relationship with our new partner begins, we become intoxicated and infatuated but if this loving energy becomes negative and dependent on the other person for our needs, we are in fact pushing that person away. It is not good to make one person the centre of our lives. We are powerful, talented, multifaceted human beings and have far-reaching abilities that makes us complete. We should not limit ourselves to depend on one person or others to fulfil us. It is not fair on us or them. Dependency on our partner and others for all our emotional needs stifles us and limits us. It is only when we can love ourselves truly from within that we can begin to set ourselves free and really learn what true love is all about.

CHAPTER 19

Longer, happier, healthier lives

We always hear about the power of positive thinking. Well, I think we should hear more about the power of laughter, fun and having the chats with our friends. The power of laughter, fun and chatting should never be underestimated. By laughing more, talking more and having more fun we are connecting with our friends, our feelings and our inner light. What a wonderful way to feel happy, by connecting with others who are like-minded, sociable and good humoured! There is nothing else like it. Meeting friends under these conditions can also make us feel loved, included and socially accepted. We can even feel we belong. We can feel we are alive. Above all, we can feel loved for being our own unique selves.

In a social setting most of us would like to feel we are:

1) included
2) belong
3) accepted

If we have these three basic feelings in our lives, we can cultivate a feeling of happiness deep within. As a result, I believe we can live longer, happier, healthier, lives.

I believe that laughter, fun, mixing with others over a meal, listening to some music and having a chat with others dispels isolation and loneliness, which are huge issues for a lot of us, including the elderly in our society. We are all going to be elderly someday; with that in mind, we need to look after our senior members of our community for their support and advice as they have survived the 'slings and arrows' of life.

Why is society divided into categories which culminates in this ageist disease? Why do we sometimes forget our elderly or those of us who are over forty? Why is there a distance within the ages thus creating ageism? How is it that the older we get, there seems to be more of a gap between the young and the old? Is it because we see our youth as the only acceptable beauty, as the only ones who are able to fund our GNP, as the only ones who are talented and the only ones important in society? Why can't we also see the beauty and grace in our beautiful, wonderful over-forties? Why can't we focus more on the beauty the rest of us have both on the outside as well as on the inside? Why can't we raise the over-forties up onto the pillar of honour and respect in our community? Maybe we need to change our perspective to include all ages especially the over-forties?

We need to make more of an effort not to exclude those over-forties because we have reached a certain age. Society, in my opinion, is misdirected to concentrate only on the youth and their physical beauty and only what they have to offer society. It is obsessional and destructive only to see beauty and ability in one category of age. We need to break the borders of ageism and accept all ages in the categories of beauty, ability and talent. We need to change our focus to what the rest of the ages have to offer such as wealth of experience, hard earned wisdom, and even harder growth lessons learned over the course of many years on this earth. Maybe if we could mix all ages together once and for all, we may learn to accept and see beauty, grace and goodness at every age? What a wonderful vision to see all ages laughing, having fun and the chats together as naturally as the air we breathe!

What do we need to do? Have you ever gone out feeling tired, but soon find that some laughter, fun and chatting in a social setting evaporates the pains and aches of life and soothes the way for a brighter day and a healthier life? We need to include everyone in our social setting, letting no one grow old alone because it is up to each and every one of us to be responsible and take care of our own.

Life is not only for the youthful who are fresh, good-looking and in their prime, it is also for all of us that don't necessarily fit into this category – we are just as beautiful, able and talented. We have just as much to offer society, if not more. But society has forgotten and become over-focused on the youth. Let us now open our eyes wide and observe what is so obvious and so important to all our well-being. Let us now concentrate on important feelings like inclusion, belonging and acceptance by everyone. We seriously need to end the divide now. We need to include, make each other feel a sense of belonging and accept each other. Our blood is all one colour.

We just have to change our perspective and learn to appreciate different types of beauty, abilities and talents at all ages, not focus on the one age category. We need to shake up our attitude and break free of the conventions that society imprisons us within to conform to this one particular physical form of beauty. It is not a healthy way to look at beauty and can be soul destroying to be rejected by society because we are not tall, skinny, young and a size six. We are not all Google mad and technology experts, but we have other things to offer – like how to survive and rebuild our lives through difficult times. It is only through difficult times that we understand the value of a close-knit community of family, friends, and neighbours.

See the vision like this: You are walking into a Spanish or Italian bar at 11pm at night. Every member of the family is around the table from the *abuelo* and *abuela* to the *bebe* is there. We need to strengthen our familial ties once again like our continental brothers and sisters.

This obsession with our youth has to change and we need to wake up to all sorts of beauty from elegance to grace, to inner beauty, to looking at kindness and gentleness as a form of beauty within all ages. We need to release the pressure valves on how people look physically. We need to relax and leave the rest of us alone to be whatever way we are meant to be, to be whatever age we are meant to be, to wear whatever we want to wear and be free to be whoever we were meant to be.

Let us get rid of the conformity to fashion trends, beauty trends and the isolation of our elderly? Can we now change our attitude and learn to mix together and share our lives together as one community? Let us learn to laugh together, have fun together, spend time together and above all, to connect as a communal family once again. The benefits are simply to live longer, happier, healthier lives.

CHAPTER 20

The real secret to success

Society deems success as material wealth and all the trappings that go with it, such as big houses, big cars, big yachts. In some cases, the people with the most amount of external wealth get the least amount of joy from this kind of wealth because real joy, peace and love comes from within.

Success is an attitude, not an object. Success in my book is self-actualisation for us, both individually and collectively. Success is about becoming who we truly really are and not about what we really have. That said, there is nothing wrong with money or material wealth. Money is just an energy we receive for transacting goods and services. Whether we are rich or poor, it all boils down to understanding our life as an experience that we chose to have on this earth. Our life on this blue planet is a pathway for our soul to grow, to learn, to develop into who we truly are.

Who are we? We are divine sparks from the source of Divine Light, from the source of divine truth, from the source of divine love. It all goes back to the source as this is where we all come from. No matter what type of person we are, good, bad, indifferent we all have a back to the source spark within us. The source spark is our journey back to our true home. This is where we will all go back to in the end. Back to the beginning.

Success is about going within and tapping into all the beauty, love, peace and joy we have been given. It is about going within and seeing the truth about ourselves and the world around us. We cannot change the world on the outside unless we change the world from the inside. We cannot change anything unless we understand what the world is truly about and where it is truly going. It is an experience we have chosen to have at this time for our soul's growth. This is a great and privileged time to be on this earth for all of us to partake in the grand ascension of Mother Earth into the fifth dimension. This is happening every day.

The effects of being raised into the fifth dimension will make life very black and white. The truth will be more apparent and more obvious. Previous grey areas will no longer be accepted. We will learn to see as clear as crystal what was previously invisible to our eyes. The obvious which was difficult to see through the smoke and mirrors of the third dimension will now be very obvious. The truth will be revealed to the world in its raw, unstained, pure fashion. We will relearn to live our truth again. This is our individual as well as our collective road to success to relearn to live our truth, in our integrity, to relearn to love one another again and to go back to the beginning.

CHAPTER 21

Turn your life around

Everything is made up of positive and negative energy. Negative energy makes us angry, agitated, even nervous. Positive energy makes us happy, relaxed and helps us cope better with the stresses and strains of life.

Five ways to keep your energy positive:

1) Protect yourself against energy vampires who dump their problems on you. Do this by imagining a gold shield around you, letting only positive energy in and out.
2) Avoid getting involved in other people's drama. Everyone has their own lessons to learn in life. This is called karma. People have to deal with their own dramas. Yes, be supportive and caring but each person has to take responsibility for their own issues individually.
3) Get outside, spend time outdoors. I know the weather is changeable but a good brisk walk along by the sea or in nature works wonders to pep up positive energy.

4) Remove emotional clutter. In doing so, we clear space in our hearts to let positive energy in to heal any pain in our lives. There is nothing wrong with a good cry and letting emotions come to the surface. After crying, turn the page and start afresh. It does the emotions a world of good.
5) Try not to overdo it in one day. The most successful people only plan fifty percent of their day. Plan to do things over the course of a week rather than squeezing everything into one day. Allow yourself time to breath. Take a power nap or meditate. There is nothing like a quick thirty-minute rest in the day to rejuvenate the batteries and balance the energies.

It is only the smallest of changes that make the biggest differences in our lives.

CHAPTER 22

Lost and unappreciated

> Have you ever felt like a spare peg in a round hole?
> Did you ever feel different and misunderstood?
> Were you ever put to one side and ignored?
> Were you ever talked at rather than talked to?
> Were you ever laughed at for not quite getting the joke?

Then you understand the feeling of exclusion, isolation, separation from the crowd like you are walking down the local main street full of people and no one can see you. No one values your uniqueness, your beauty, your smile, your sense of humour, your opinion – no one values you. Instead, they brush past you like you are invisible, forgotten like the lost people of Atlantis. All rushing around in their busy lives doing important things. But what is more important than another human being? Someone, who you can share a greeting with, someone who you can share the acknowledgement of your existence, someone who you can share a passing moment or some common civility like 'Good Morning! How are you?' and really meaning it.

How do we make ourselves feel loved and valued, and not lost and unappreciated?

Firstly, all feelings whether positive or negative come from inside us and if we can balance the positive and negative energy in our bodies, we can learn to accept and increase our self-worth and this can be done through spiritual healing, for example.

Secondly, we need to go within, look at ourselves, accept and understand how perfect each one of us really is. We need to learn to see ourselves as not being Hollywood's so-called perfect size six, perfect hair, perfect teeth and perfect skin. We need to learn to see that Hollywood's external beauty requirements are not real and as we know, they come at a very high price. We need to accept that we are not all made to order. We need to accept that we are all different shapes and sizes and that these differences make us stand apart from each other. We need to accept without any doubt our very own genuine inner beauty. No one can take that away from us. No other person is me. No other person looks exactly like me. So, by accepting ourselves, it means accepting all of us and understanding that each of our unique differences from one another is in actual fact perfection at the highest level.

Thirdly, we need to learn to value and love ourselves before we can ask another human being to appreciate and see us as one of a kind. Valuing and loving ourselves from within is the key against feelings of being lost and unappreciated. Loving that no one else has got a smile quite like ours, loving that no one else has a personality quite like ours, loving that no one else understands the world quite the way we do and that no one else has quite the same opinion as us. We therefore need to value ourselves as being real and authentic individuals before others can love us the way we need to be loved.

Fourthly, we can say affirmations to ourselves such as the following:

I am responsible for loving and accepting myself.

I am responsible for how I feel about myself.

I am responsible for my own inner belief.

I am responsible for accepting myself as I am at this present moment and no one else.

The fact that we are all packaged differently should be celebrated and not lamented. We are not all the same. Fact! Why do we want to be the same as everyone else anyway? Why do we want to be sheep?

Finally, if you have experienced and can answer in the affirmative to all the above four questions at the top of this article than you are no sheep. You are a special, rare, and beautiful individual with looks and talents no one else has. You just have to be able to reinforce that belief in yourself. Give yourself the gift of being free to be yourself. Give yourself the gift of loving yourself and not feeling guilty. Give yourself the gift of accepting who you really are and enjoying every step of the journey. Instead of being lost and unappreciated, you will bring into being a rare and wonderful person living life to its fullest.

CHAPTER 23

21/12/2012

Many scaremongers among us believed this to be the day the world was going to end, but to many energy healers, it signified the world being re-started.

The Earth, also called Gaia (mother nature), was undergoing a major re-birth. Gaia was shifting a lot of the negative energies built up over thousands of years, especially throughout the last two centuries, when man has not been kind to the earth. Man has extracted her minerals, bombed her, polluted her, caused global warming, created acid rain, destroyed her through deforestation and the list goes on.

The reason why Gaia was getting ready for a re-birth is that the planet was undergoing a transition from the Age of Pisces to the new Age of Aquarius on the 21/12/2012. Many energy healers believed this transition to be a positive step for mankind. Gaia was re-awakening from a long slumber, preparing for a spiritual uplifting of her energies then. They believed also that mankind would undergo a physical and spiritual awakening. It simply meant that life would be better with more positive experiences happening to us than negative ones. Mankind has a been given a second chance to awaken his energies once again.

CHAPTER 24

Be happy

Where do we find happiness?

Happiness is not a destination. It is not a place where we can go. It is not something that we can buy. It is something that we can develop and grow from within. We can find happiness by examining our attitude to life. An attitude can be positive or negative. An attitude is a choice that we can make on how we want to look at things in life. It is an outlook that we acquire over a period of time, but we don't just suddenly wake up and have an attitude or be happy.

The attitude grows and grows throughout our lives until it takes hold like the roots of an oak tree. The tree can be shaken and stirred, go through the four seasons of life but the roots remain firm and can go deep within the earth like the roots of happiness grow deep within us. We can aim to plant a positive attitude within our mindset and then the attitude creates positive feelings of contentment, joy, peace and we eventually over time achieve a very fertile plateau of happiness.

How can we feel happy all the time?

Now we know there are dark moments, dark days and dark feelings but the more we develop our attitude, the quicker the feeling of contentment comes back, and the feeling of happiness just exists within us. The oak trees do not always look like a fully grown oak tree. It went through years of growth and change to adapt to all weathers. Adapting a positive attitude towards all dilemmas gets us through in life.

It is by learning a survival attitude to all crises in life that we survive. Our attitude then creates a feeling of peace no matter what happens to us. We can see beyond the immediate problem or pain and we know that all will be fine. We will take the positive out of every situation. We learn to think and see everything in life as a gift, that all situations do and will turn around for the greater good.

Do people make us happy?

We don't acquire happiness through superficial relationships and material wealth because happiness is a decision we make from within. Learning to see every crisis as a lesson and a gift from the universe, will make us stronger, wiser and better people. Knowing that life is not about having problems but rather accepting them as part of the deal, just like the conditions in a contract. Life may just simplify itself. We know that problems and dilemmas just don't go away, unfortunately. We must know and understand that we are here on this beautiful earth to find out who we really are and that without our challenges, we wouldn't grow into the beings we are meant to be and learn the lessons we are meant to learn. Then we will find the right path.

Let's look at happiness as a belief that everything is for our greater good and will work out for the best in the end. It is a consciousness. It is an awareness of self. It is an awareness of who we really are, why we are here and where we are going as one complete global community.

CHAPTER 25

Ego vs heart

Are you controlled by your lower self?
Are you dominated by the voice of your inner child?
Are you more secular than spiritual?
Are you afraid of being spiritual?

There are two parts to the self – the higher self and the lower self. The higher self is connected to our spiritual growth and the lower self is connected to our secular growth. When we keep our energies within our lower self then we live in the world of our ego, our personality and our inner child. We become people of the mind, we are cold, intellectual and very controlling.

We try to judge people and control the outcome of every situation. We want everything our own way. We also have an over-inflated belief in our own opinion, and we are always right. We will defy any other way but our own way. We believe in status, in fear, and in being the victim. Our ego dominates our world and those around us because we are afraid to let go and raise our energies to a higher level.

When our energies are connected to the higher self, we are connected to our heart and we believe that every situation is for our highest good, regardless of the outcome. We live in the world of unconditional love. We show compassion. We are sharing and caring. We are willing to change for the good of everyone around us. We are warm, empathetic, kind and self-confident. We have our own self power, and we are balanced.

We have self-respect and protect ourselves by placing boundaries around ourselves. We don't believe in failure, as we learn from everything we do. We have self-admiration, self-confidence, self-glorification, self-love, self-regard, self-satisfaction, self-sufficiency, self-trust, self-worth, and self-sufficiency. We believe in ourselves. We love ourselves. We know we are perfect. We know we are protected and guided by the universe. We know we are responsible for the quality of love and happiness in our life. We know we are responsible for the people we accept into our lives. We know the people with whom to maintain friendship with and whom to let go. We forgive people for not being what we want them to be. We know we can create the life that we want to create.

If we move from concentrating on the old, outdated, repetitive thoughts in our mind and listen to the pure, positive, pulses of the heart, we can make life-changing decisions for the good of ourselves and those around us. If we move our energies from the lower self to the higher self, we can make far-reaching changes – not only in our own personal world but also in our outer world. We can live a life of peace and unity. We can learn to live as one.

CHAPTER 26

To judge or not to judge

Do you attack people before they attack you?
Do you put people on the defence?
Do you put people into boxes?
Do you ignore people before they ignore you?
Do you pre-judge people or do you accept them?

If we all understand that there is no right or wrong that there just is, the world would be a much less complicated place. If we didn't split the world into two camps of right and wrong and we saw all our experiences as lessons, how much easier would it not all be for us to accept each other? If we looked at the world as one complete unit rather than as separated into sections – like continents, countries, counties, communities – how much more simplified would our perception of everything be?

During a visit to the Vatican in Rome, I told a priest my views on right and wrong, that my sins were just lessons and he refused to absolve me from my sins. The absolver became the judge and jury of my life's journey. If we could all believe that we are here to further our path of enlightenment, to learn to become better people, then why do we have preconceived notions about people? Why do we assume or pre-judge people without any grounds or evidence because of their beliefs, attitudes and actions?

If we could believe in a basic code of ethics and hold value judgements based on our core worth rather than holding pre-judgements based on assumptions, then we would be free of inequality, injustice and intolerance. Hatred, horror and hostility would be transmuted into charity, compassion and community. We would all have much simpler lives and have much simpler relationships with others.

If we could compare judgement to a crown of thorns and could see judgement like an affliction that causes great suffering, it would make us think twice about piercing another person with the long wooden spiny stems of our words, presumptions, presuppositions and pure pain? If we could throw down our crown of thorns and avoid making stinging, scourging prejudices, could we learn to wear the wreath of victory and tolerance, learn to respect and recognize the beliefs and practices of others?

CHAPTER 27

Money attitude

There are three types of attitudes:

1) The Las Vegas type
2) The Edinburgh type
3) The Italian Riviera type

1) The Las Vegas type attitude to money.

This is the gambler type attitude. The attitude is feckless, fickle, and flighty with money. They are unaccountable, unanswerable, and above all, unpredictable. Along with this attitude they just don't care about anyone, anything or the outcome.

There are two sides to their personality. The giver and the taker. They are the giver when they are out in their casino. They are the giver when they are in their Imperial Palace Hotel. Sitting at the head of the crap table is like sitting on their very own throne. They are the king and the world bows to their every whim because they have money, and they like to throw it around to show how kind and generous they are.

Las Vegas types go through cycles of having plenty of money and then being absolutely broke. Typical characteristics of how they spend money are: it burns a whole in their pocket and they just can't get rid of it quick enough, as spending money is the only thing which gives them that ultimate high. They keep putting money into their one-armed bandit until it's gone. Money fixes everything. Once they have money, they are the king of the joint, untouchable, they love everyone, and everyone loves them. Their energies are high and addictive as they can pull people into their space and everyone gets in on the buzz. They are so charming, so funny that they become the life and soul of the place. We could never meet a nicer person on that night in that mood.

But then the cycle goes from boom to bust. They have a riches to rags mentality.

Now the low comes. The mood changes from the generous giver, to the towering taker that knows no ends. They become a scrounger. They need to borrow money to survive. They have to live like paupers until their pay packet comes around again. The rich-to-poor cycle continues over and over again, over each month, over each year, perhaps throughout their whole lifetimes. They continually moan and groan that they cannot afford to do anything, buy anything, everything is so expensive. They play Russian Roulette with the bills. Money is their obsession. Having money in their eyes gives them a value. They have to have money as this is how they measure their own self-worth.

Without money they become insecure, difficult, even negative. Where once they were the king, now they are the pauper. They have no self-worth or value for anything else without money.

Their energies change too now. They pollute the house with their darkened mood. They are in a dark place and they want us to be in their black hole with them. We cannot go anywhere in peace during this time because if the Las Vegas type can't be happy, they will do their best to make sure you are definitely not.

2) The Edinburgh type attitude to money.

This is a negative attitude. They are the miser, the saver, the scrooge. They only ever have one mood. One that is severe, sour and stringent. One that is hard, harsh and always unhappy about something. They have to be in full control on the inside as well as on the outside. The have to control their environment. Once they have the control of the money, they are in control of their environment and everyone around them. Everything comes down to money. Money is their God.

Their personality is cold, tight-fisted and selfish. They are someone who if they had two euro, would save one euro. Thriftiness is a religion, a way of life. Their attitude, mood, and personality are always the same. There are no two sides to their personality as there is with the Las Vegas type. They are mean and cold-hearted. They will always find a cheaper way to save money. They will always keep to their budget. They will always have loads of little piggy banks for saving even the smallest of change. They hoard money. Money in the bank is their security and their power. With money, they are God, and we know it.

Typical characteristics of the Edinburgh type is they don't like spending money and they don't like to see other people spending money either. They will always tell us where we went wrong in our budget. They will always tell us to turn off the light, turn off the heat and put on another jumper if we are feeling cold. They have no generous Christmas spirit. They are always in Lent, always denying themselves any comfort. They are always despising and humbugging anything that makes other people happy.

They have a poverty mentality nothing every satisfies them. Nothing is ever good enough for them no matter how much money they get. No matter how much time and attention are given to them, they always want more. They are always dissatisfied. They are always in want of something or somebody.

They are energy vampires. They sap every last particle of energy from our souls. They steal, store and stockpile energy from others.

3) The Italian Riviera type attitude to money.

This is a positive attitude and is all about a 'having it all' attitude. They know they are worth it. They know they are spectacular just like the beautiful landscape of the Riviera. They know they are as dazzling as the magnificent coastline. They have all they need in their lives. They have abundance. They have everything. They take responsibility for the quality of their own lives.

Their personalities are like the climate – well-balanced. They have always got money at the end of the month because they know their own value. They know their own beauty. They know that like the villages on the Riviera, they have charm, sophistication and uniqueness. They would have no hesitation in sharing, giving and receiving. They are never the underdog because they know their own self-worth.

They respect and love themselves enough to have a price on their time, on their work and on their efforts in life. They have all their boundaries clearly defined. If they do something for another person, they expect that person to return the favour without guilt or feeling under compliment. People with this attitude have an abundant mentality as they are always satisfied with everything they have in their life as they always have enough.

The Italian Riviera types' energies are bountiful. They know how to protect their energies from the negative vampires. They know how to only allow love, life and laughter into their lives. They are never in a dark place because they know how to avoid getting into it. Their sun shines day and night. They abound with abundance in everything.

Finally, the universe only knows abundance. The universe gives us exactly what we ask for. When we take on the attitude of abundance, as in the Italian Riviera attitude, we can manifest great changes and riches into our lives, but we alone are responsible for those changes. We alone are responsible for the quality of our own lives and yes, it is alright to have an easy life.

CHAPTER 28

A truly successful life

Do we know our core values?

Here are some core examples:

Integrity	Self-Reliance	Optimism
Truth	Strength	Originality
Trust	Intuition	Independence
Love	Empathy	Making a difference

The most successful people on the planet make a personal growth plan regularly by making a list of their core values with the intention of growing their inner personal worth and confidence. To do this we need to choose values that sounds like our character.

There are many reasons for knowing our core values. They will help us know and value our own self-worth. They will help us make better decisions in our lives and help us understand our attitude to people by showing us whether we like them or not, can work with them or not, or can have a relationship with them or not.

Do we know who we truly are?

Another reason for knowing our core values is that they are central to our core identity, of who we are. If we do not know ourselves and know what we are about, we leave ourselves open to creating a false identity, a false image of ourselves which we put on for our equally false friends. If we create a false image of ourselves, we lose touch with who we truly are, and we lose touch with our inner barometer of uniqueness. If we have to portray a false image to others, we can suppress our emotions of how we really feel about the superficial people in our lives. We lose ourselves in a myriad of falsity and lose our true inner connection to ourselves and most of all, we lose our true inner connection to the genuine people in our lives.

Do we value our own personal time enough?

We can spend too much time with the wrong people and not enough time with the real people in our lives. We need to be true to ourselves, to who we really are. We need to learn not to portray a certain learned image to humour other people. We do not need to dress in a certain way in certain clothes, with certain hairstyles and follow a certain way of life. We do not need to depend on our external image and other people's reactions to us. The secret to strong inner values is being true to ourselves because if we are only concerned with superficial values, we are vulnerable to losing who we genuinely are, and we are susceptible to peer pressure from all sectors of life. We do not need to let others shape our identity as we are the masters of our own identity.

Do we hide how we really feel?

Yet another reason for knowing our values is for when we suppress them – we deny what we truly feel on the inside whilst on the outside we portray all is well and perfect. We lose touch with our own inner alarm of well-being as our emotions explain to us how we are coping whether we are sad, depressed or happy.

Our emotional barometer is then faulty and in need of repair. If we don't understand how others affect us or make us feel, we can find it hard to be comfortable in other people's company. If we are with people who have different core values to us, we may find that we will clash with them and that misunderstandings will constantly arise. It is therefore advisable that we choose friends, colleagues and most of all, a long-term partner who has the same basic values as ourselves.

Do we protect ourselves from others?

Our inner core values dictate how we can react to other people and situations. Our core values protect our identity, provide us with boundaries and limits of how we should be treated and how we react. If someone threatens our core values, they are not being respectful or understanding to us and are not valuing our self-worth. When someone does that, it should not be taken too lightly. Friends, family, etc. should know or if not, we should tell them that they are crossing the line and disrespecting our very own personal code of conduct and even though we may choose to forgive this time, generally this behaviour is not acceptable, and it insults our inner core of who we are and how we live our lives. This is a basic human right and the basis of true freedom. Uniqueness and originality should be enhanced and encouraged not manipulated and mistreated.

Do we really want to be successful?

If we do not align ourselves to our inner core values, we will find it hard to be successful because our values dictate to us how we live our lives, how we act, what we say and what we think. If our values are strong, then no one can sway us away from our own standards and principals. We find this with very successful people who derive great inner strength, especially through adversity, by knowing who they are and what they are about. As they live their lives according to their own inner core of personal values and beliefs, that is the secret to their success.

CHAPTER 29

The road to happiness

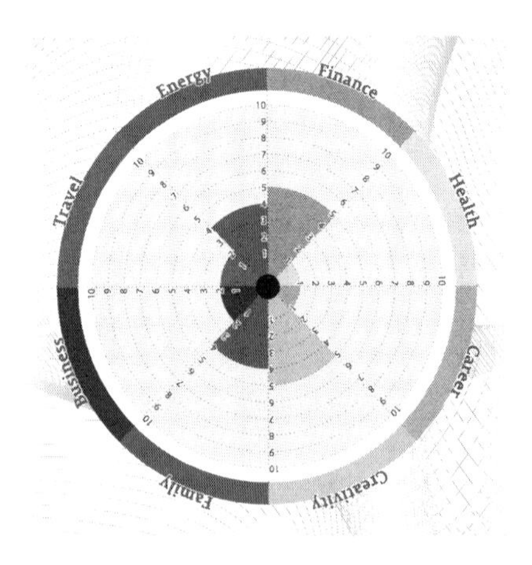

Is your life all work and no play?

Are you living the life you want to live?

Are you the person who you really want to be?

Are all the areas in your life balanced or unbalanced?

Very successful people always look as if they have it all. How is that possible? How can we have it all too? The wheel of life is a good indicator to show us if our life is balanced or unbalanced, too focused on one area and not focused enough in another area. If we spend most of our time working long hours, all the other areas in our lives such as our family, our partner, our health, our social life become out of sync and neglected.

Too much focus in one area means that we lack focus in other areas. The German saying *alles in maßen* especially rings true. It means 'everything in moderation' and as many successful people believe, is the golden solution to the success and happiness in their lives. Another reason to find balance in our lives is that we are not machines, we are human beings with many gifts and talents. We need to develop and grow in all sections of our lives to be who we want to be and live the life we are all here to live.

The above wheel of life shows examples of areas we find important in our lives, but they can be different for each individual depending on what he/she believes to be vital in his/her life. Once we have picked the vital areas, the idea then is to score with a pen from one (low) to ten (high) our focus of attention in each segment at this moment in our lives. The score can change in each segment as we focus on different things at different stages in our lives. Now we need to link the scores together with a pen and see if our lives are in balance.

If one or two areas dominate, it is time to rethink and rejig our focus to find a better balance. The same rings true for areas which are not receiving any attention at all. The idea is not to draw a perfect circle or have perfect tens but to show areas where we can redress the imbalance.

Once we have finished that, the next thing we need to do is to write in our ideal scores and then link them again to show a more balanced wheel of life. This can be our aim for the year ahead. It may be better to concentrate on one or two areas at a time rather than trying to improve all areas at once.

The main idea is that, as human beings, we always need positive goals, as well as a purpose so that we can strive to have more rewarding, happier, successful lives.

CHAPTER 30

Real love

Do we love conditionally, or do we love unconditionally?

Have we become such a consumer society that we now see people like a product on a shelf? Do we see people like something that fulfils a need and only want a person when they can give us something to satisfy that need, whether it's money, a job, a house, a car, pay the bills, a baby and once their sell buy date is up we just get another product to match our needs? Is that it?

Have we become so insatiable that our needs are like a bottomless pit never ever getting enough, always wanting more and more? We are all becoming like economic goods, ready for consumption by the masses. We are all out there in the factory of life as something to be bought, used and discarded because once we are consumed, we are considered to be of no use. We are then immediately removed from the economic conveyor belt of life and thrown in the trash.

In such a society, where does love fit in? If we base our love on what others can give us, seeing others as filling our empty cavern of endless needs and wants, then this can cause heavy dependency on others and the love we are actually sharing is based on the condition that our needs are met. This is called conditional love because it's based on all our needs been satisfied. However, once our needs are not met, we move on to the next person to fulfil our never-ending needs and our forever unsatisfied nagging desires.

What if we learned to meet our own needs and be independent, detach by standing on our own two feet? What if we learned to become self-sufficient in the magical, serene flow of life? We may then try and learn to discipline our needs and take control by not allowing them to control us or enslave us. We are on the ever-demanding conveyor belt of needs that never stops moving because our needs force us to depend on others. We experience things we would not necessarily experience if we freed ourselves from our and their needs and wants.

What if we learned detachment from material things, emotional needs and physical desires? We can then free ourselves to live in the universal flow of life where there is no need to live by other people's rules or conditions and for this effort we slowly learn to love unconditionally. We learn to be free mentally, emotionally and physically. We learn to free ourselves from others and they free themselves from us. We learn the power of choice. We learn to have the strength to be with others for who they really are and not for what we can get. We eventually learn unconditional love for ourselves and for others.

This means we learn to really take care of ourselves and others out of free will and not out of any need or desire to acquire something from them to fulfil our endless, spiralling out of control wants and needs. We learn peace, calmness and kindness all over again, in their true state and purest form. We break free from the chains of dependency.

We break free from the ropes of compulsion strangling us to get our needs met over and over again. We become free from the whips and lashes of bitterness and pain because we are no longer slaves to other people or ourselves. We learn self-mastery and we learn to come into our own and reach our fullest potential. We learn to live again and find our true purpose, which is to unconditionally love ourselves and others.

Finally, unconditional love of self comes first and then we can learn to unconditionally love others. Unconditional love is a state of truth. Unconditional love is a state of perfection in its purest form. Unparalleled to any other emotional, mental or physical state we could ever experience. This is the true purpose of humanity. This is our true goal and this why we are here.

CHAPTER 31

Stress

Why do we allow ourselves to be over-stressed?
Why do we allow ourselves to be over-worked?
Why do we allow ourselves to be over-emotional?
Why do we allow ourselves to be over-tired?

Why can we not see ourselves as fragile, vulnerable, soft, sensitive human beings? Why can't we see that we are we are not robots, machines or metal objects? Why can't we see ourselves as gentle, kind, sincere human beings made out of flesh and blood? We bleed. We cry. We hurt. We get nervous. We get scared. We feel alone. We feel misunderstood. We feel unappreciated. Why is this? The reason for this is because we have lost our way, we have forgotten who we are, we have forgotten why we are here and where we are going.

How do we protect a newborn baby from the rain, the cold, the frost, the wind, too much sun, the hazards of the elements? We wrap it up and we talk gently to it, we kiss it softly, we protect it with our heart and soul. We kindle the helpless child with all our love. So why do we forget to do this to ourselves when we grow up? We are still that soul, we are still that person, we just look different.

Newborn babies need love, they need to be looked after, their beauty appreciated and so do we. Why does all that stop? Why do we forget to care for ourselves? What do we need to do? We need to give ourselves time to bloom, time to flourish, time to excel and time to be in our prime.

But how can we be at our best when we are stressed, over-tired, over-worked, and when we are over-emotional? What do we need to do? We need to go within and listen to ourselves and let our true nature come to the fore. We need to give ourselves time to discover our authentic selves and time to be still and quiet. We need to listen to our inner voice without the noise of the outside world.

This year let's give ourselves a present of some down time, to relax, time to think, to be on our own. We will reap the benefits.

CHAPTER 32

Less stress

Slow down

Over the year, do we ever give ourselves a few minutes to breathe and just take some time out? No, we don't. Instead, we rush and race around to get everything done and then when every piece of energy has evaporated, we collapse into the chair unable to move for hours. Is that you? Well, maybe if we slowed it all down and took some time out to breathe instead of overloading ourselves by pushing and pushing to get everything done, we would then make our year, our life a lot easier for ourselves and others.

Simplify our schedule

Do we have too many events, friends and places to visit this year? Do we put ourselves under so much pressure to be somewhere? Do we expect so much of ourselves that we just don't have time to appreciate what we are doing and who we are meeting? Yes, we do, because we haven't time to think. We are rushing so quickly onto the next event, meeting the next person, visiting the next place that we haven't time to do anything else but collapse.

What can we do?

The secret is to plan ahead and do half as much in a day rather than more. Simplifying our schedule is better than overcrowding it. How come? By simplifying our schedule and allowing plenty of time between events, we allow ourselves to take time out to breathe and gather ourselves if things get too hectic.

Secondly, by giving ourselves plenty of time we allow for things go pear-shaped – such as needing extra time when we forgot to wrap a present for a friend we are meeting or when needing extra cash before going to a party and we have to wait forever at the cash point! We will have no cause for concern because we will have already thought of that by allowing ourselves plenty of extra time before meeting our friends or before going to that party.

Thirdly, planning activities over the week so as when shopping, if a present can't be bought at a certain time, we know it can be carried forward to the next day or later on in the week. This avoids extra pressure and stress on any particular day. So, now let's just try to enjoy every minute of our time by simplifying rather than overcrowding our day. Let's stop rushing onto the next event, person or place. Let's just learn to enjoy the moment one step at a time. We can learn to adjust to less chaos and stress in our lives by simplifying it and making life much easier by doing less instead of more. Hence making our life a much more enjoyable one.

Saving energy

The secret to getting things done during the year is as easy as already stated – learn to plan! This saves hours of chaos and stress. But planning our lists and pacing ourselves to get everything done in plenty of time also saves our much-needed energy. Instead of rushing around like headless chickens, flying around in a panic, running from queue to queue, from checkout to checkout, from shop to shop killing ourselves to have everything done by a certain time, think of all the energy we are using up and the stress we are enduring.

Please stop before this happens. Take time out to plan the days ahead. Sit down, plan, pace and prepare all the things we have to do in advance. Ensure this includes taking regular breaks and allows plenty of time out to breathe, to rejuvenate enough energy to give ourselves the chance to enjoy all the excitement in our lives and making our lives much less stressful and chaotic.

Stop worrying

Worrying kills the enjoyment of the moment. 99% of what we worry about never happens. But we spend most our time thinking of all the things that may go wrong instead of thinking of the lovely experiences that may go right. By not worrying, we can give ourselves peace of mind and find ourselves actually really looking forward to living rather than dreading it because we are just too exhausted, overloaded and wishing it was all over so we can get back to normal.

How about trying and trusting that everything will work out for the better? Instead of worrying, think of the funny side of it all and try not taking it all so seriously. So what if something goes wrong? It is not the end of the world. Sometimes when things go wrong, they make great stories to tell around the dinner table and everyone can have a good laugh. So please change the worrying channel to the chilled and trusting channel because this will definitely make life easier and much more fun.

Sleeping more

We all know how ratty we can be without a good night sleep. Let's give ourselves loads of relaxation time to have plenty of rest and good nights' sleep before any parties and nights out get underway. When we are fresh and rested, we look and feel better.

It is well worthwhile to get to bed earlier, chill out and have plenty of rest so we can really make the most of making everyones' lives easier and more enjoyable. Remember to switch off all those mobile devices when sleeping so as not to disrupt your sleep. There is nothing worse than a disturbed sleep. Get plenty of rest and sleep to ease our way through a peaceful year.

CHAPTER 33

For Christmas

What would you like for Christmas?

Why not ask for a special gift for the entire world?

Well, how about asking Santa for the gift of gratitude? Gratitude is the greatest gift we will ever receive this Christmas. Why is it so great? It is so great because gratitude is an eternal gift, which tunes into the Christmas stocking of abundance.

In the hustle and bustle of life do we really mean the words 'thank you' when we say it? Little do we know that these two words are so precious and powerful that if Santa asked us what gift we would like to give to our family, our friends and our community this Christmas, we ought to be without a doubt ask for the gift of gratitude.

Why is gratitude so important? Gratitude is very important because once we tune into the universal wavelength of gratitude, we tap into its magical treasure trove of gorgeous presents and gifts. Just like Santa, there is nothing that the universe won't give to us. All we have to do is simply open our hearts, say what we need, say our wants and desires, and absolutely believe that whatever comes in our path is for our greater good no matter what. We must hold on and trust that the universe is really like Santa's Christmas grotto – full of magic, tinsel and fairy lights that our special wishes are truly at the universes command.

To really tune into the cheerful merriment of abundance, all we must do is show our gratitude for all our blessings, achievements, possessions, beautiful towns, lovely countryside, the people in our lives and above all, our beloved planet. The more that gratitude grows in our nature, the more the universe wants to shower us with everything we need. We just have to trust and be patient.

When we overflow with angelic spirit of magical gratitude, we overflow like the warm, spicy, mulled wine in our crystal glass of life. We then slowly change from within and our whole world gradually begins to change around us, and all our dreams eventually become manifested for us, our families and for the greater good. So, as you see, by switching on the Christmas lights of gratitude and shining its light wherever we go, we are able to spread love, peace and joy on earth. Isn't that what Christmas is all about?

What an amazing gift we'd give ourselves by spreading love, peace and joy throughout our lives and throughout our whole world without any cost involved. All by saying two simple words – Thank you. Thank you. Thank you. It really is that simple.

This Christmas let's give ourselves the gift of gratitude allowing abundance to sprout from every core of our being by growing and manifesting a world where we are all accepted, we are all loved and where we all feel we belong. At this special time of year, let's awaken the spirit of Christmas in our hearts and share goodwill to all by showing gratitude for everything and everyone we have in our lives.

Thank you for your time.
Happy Christmas to one and all.

CHAPTER 34

Inclusion or invisible barriers

As we begin anew, let's look ahead and ponder whether inclusiveness is all-inclusive, or are there still invisible barriers in our community and society?

The word inclusiveness is thankfully everywhere, which is very enlightening and embracing. At last, we are now calling on our gay, lesbian, transgender brothers and sisters, our differently abled, our elderly – we are calling on everyone to be accepted into the fold of the community. Society is just so amazing and wonderful.

But have we forgotten one simple little thing?

Have we forgotten the most important word in the dictionary of life, a word which we may find incredibly difficult to say and even more difficult to carry out?

What is that word, I hear you ask. The word is forgiveness. Lack of forgiveness may just be one of the biggest invisible barriers to an all-inclusive community and enriched society in the world, as we know it today.

In Al Anon when dealing with addictive natures, they say to learn to separate the addiction from the person. Can we perhaps also apply this concept to other situations too? Can we not learn to separate the mistakes and hurts of our parents, partners, children, friends, in the same way as in Al Anon when we are asked to separate the destructive force of addictiveness to the person? Let me make myself clear.

In Al Anon we are asked to still see the addict as a human being and treat him/her with human dignity and respect, despite any hurt or pain we may be feeling inside or that they may have caused us. If we apply this to others, can we learn to treat our fellow members of our family, community and society as human beings regardless of their destructive natures and their differences?

Yes, we can but why should we do this as don't they deserve all that's coming to them for the pain and suffering they caused? For one thing, we are all getting older and life is brief and transient. We need to remind ourselves over and over again that we are only here for a short time.

Let no one grow old alone. Whatever our past failings or our misunderstandings, we are all human. We are all frail. We are all sensitive. We all make many mistakes. If we could see the act of forgiveness as an amazing gift to ourselves and others, could we also learn that forgiveness is the secret and bonding effect to the unity of any community and society in general?

In our reaction to difficult and painful experiences, we learn over time to avoid and blame others for things we don't understand until we find ourselves in similar situations. Then and only then, can we empathise with our parents, siblings or friends. Maybe, we even find it's too late and they have passed on. If this is not the case, then let us reflect and think of how lucky we are to still have our family members and our friends around us to embrace us in our entirety – warts and all.

We now have the opportunity to make up. We now have the time to sort things out. We still have time to show we care because this is how we build a strong family. This is how we build an all-inclusive community where no one grows old alone.

Now more than ever, is the time to break down the invisible barriers of a divided community because by forgiving and forgetting the past battles and hurts of life, we learn acceptance of each other. We know, oh yes, we know that this is not going to be easy. But it is possible over time to accept that our parents, our siblings and most of all that we, ourselves, are but human and that we are all prone to huge errors and destructive actions.

Eventually we might see and learn how the act of forgiveness is so very vital to us. How about starting by trying to forgive ourselves for our past mistakes, our mis-judgments, our misunderstandings and our crazy actions. Then secondly, forgive others. If we don't, then how can we learn to develop, grow as individuals and grow as a collective if we are judged, isolated and rejected from the family, community and society as a whole?

We all deserve second chances. We all deserve to be given the chance to rebuild bridges and if we can try and put our worst nightmares down to experience, we can learn to build on what we learned and turn any difficult situation into an opportunity for growth and development in our own lives, relationships and communities.

Forgiveness is the golden key to acceptance, which opens the door to an all-embracing inclusive society and community. With the action of forgiveness, we bring our nearest and dearest back into the fold, our open arms, our family circle and our community. As a result of our actions, we become surrounded by our loved ones, our pillars of support, our beacons of light, shining their love on our winding, long path ahead but now we are not alone, and we will never again be alone because we are surrounded by them.

Finally, if we really want to build an all-inclusive, embracing society, we have to look at the invisible barriers. Those barriers which block all our paths no matter who we are, no matter how old we are. Above all, in order to lay the foundations for an all-inclusive society, we need to learn to forgive, forget and embrace each other. It may take time. It may take years, but it can happen. Time is a great healer, enabling us to remove those invisible barriers making way for a strong community and vibrant society once again.

Maybe this is the way forward.

CHAPTER 35

Acceptance

Part 1

Why are there things in life we cannot change?
How do we survive the pain of tragedy?
How do we love again?

The greatest and worst experiences in our lives always, always, have great love and great pain perfectly interwoven like a sailors white knot plaited tightly together into those unforgettable, life-changing events that torture us, shape us and make us who we are.

Great love and great pain are feelings we firstly have to experience and live through before we can learn to accept them. This may take many years of reflection. We need plenty of time and support before we can unplait the knot of pain that we're feeling. It is only in hindsight that we can recognise the love that was all around us, soothing the rope burns of pain, helping us push through the darkness.

We will find that with every great pain comes even greater love from amazing people who shield us and help us through the dark times. These experiences can bring us closer together as a family and as a community. Shared pain tightens the bond of love to help us through.

If we could only have the mindset during our darkest days that maybe today is our day to cry but our time will come when it will be our day to love and laugh again. If we could understand during our darkest hour that the great experiences of life are a cycle. If we could look at it that sometimes our experiences are a cycle of pain. At other times, our experiences are a cycle of love that happens throughout the course of our lives. It happens not only to us but to everyone we know. No one is free from experiencing great love and great pain.

As we get older, we try to accept and understand that dark days too shall pass. We try to help each other through the darkness of tragedy which slowly brings us back to the light again. But these things can happen more than once. Then we are back to the darkness and once again, we find ourselves picking ourselves up and returning to the light but always, always remember where there is great pain, there is also great love and even greater miracles to behold.

Part 2

How does true acceptance work and is it the greatest gift of all?

How do we get to the stage of acceptance?

Do we cry our way to acceptance by experiencing the death of our children, wives, parents, brothers, sisters and friends?

> Are there stages of acceptance or is acceptance the outcome of the grieving process?

These are questions we may ask ourselves over and over again. Learning acceptance, learning that pain and love are intermingled throughout the course of our whole lives from cradle to grave, and that as we grow older the pain doesn't get any easier, but we learn to accept that there are days of great pain but not to forget that there are also days of great love? If only it was that simple and logical but maybe it's worth reflecting upon.

We know that the love for our children, spouse, family and friends and their love for us keeps the adrenalin of life pumping through our veins. The kindness, generosity and patience of the people around us keeps the blood of life flowing through our hearts, keeping the heartbeat pulsating, helping us through the long cumbersome days of pain.

However, something inside may inspire us to know that acceptance might be the key to harmony in every torturous situation we find ourselves in.

In the dark days, we wonder how it is possible to accept the tragic experiences like the untimely death of our loved ones, terminal illnesses, poverty, homelessness. Maybe just maybe if we understood and learned acceptance, it would help us somehow through our darkest days and nights. Maybe if we had an understanding that nothing is fixed, that every moment in time is transient, that this pain too shall pass and yes, there are better days to come, we would cope better.

Acceptance of all feelings – whether of love or of pain, may be the key to finding the gift of acceptance and that both feelings are inevitable in the course of our lives. But by learning acceptance, we then gradually find the cure for mending our broken hearts. This provides us with the medicine to continue on through the interwoven twists and bends of life. Learning acceptance can also let us know that we can help others who find themselves in the same dark situations we found ourselves in. Shared pain bonds us all forever.

Acceptance plus the support of those travelling with us on our journey, can be the driving force to help us get up every morning to face the day. We can all help each other to continue and survive the endless pang of pain burning in our hearts. But love for each other is the petrol in our bloodstream that keeps us motoring forwards, even at a very low speed. Every tiny step each day is progress.

Part 3

Does our life only begin when the pain of loss seeps through every pore of our being? When the pain of failure, bankruptcy, or the pain of ill health raise their ugly heads in our lives? Should we look at it as being our beginning, our beginning of why we are truly here?

Maybe it's through pain and love we learn the lessons of life making us who we truly are, making us who we are truly meant to be which is a higher version, our true selves.

We are all mirrors of each other, both in love and in pain, swirling around in the pot noodle of life – sometimes we're in hot water and sometimes we're not. Acceptance does not stop the pain, but it provides us with the soothing ointment to heal the wound, but the scar will always be there as a reminder of our humanity, vulnerability and fragility.

Reminders that we are all only here for a short time and with the help of those remaining, allow the beautiful rose of acceptance to grow in our hearts and souls and to be handed down to the children who will learn too to pass the torch of acceptance on to the younger generation coming behind them.

Acceptance that love and pain are intertwined in all our lives is a great legacy to leave our loved ones. Handing down the torch of acceptance is the light of future hope and a valuable gift to help us continue on our journey together and for all generations to come.

CHAPTER 36

The emotional line

Do you know how to prevent others from walking over you?
Do you own your emotions?
Do you bury them to keep the peace?

Some emotions lend themselves to being expressed at the moment they happen, such as the positive emotions of compassion, love, joy, happiness, empathy. But it's a different situation when it comes to other emotions, such as crying or showing we are upset. Why are we made feel awkward when we want to share our pain, grief or anxiety with our family and friends? Don't we need them to help us through the darkness? Why are we so uncomfortable with showing these emotions? Why are others uncomfortable with us releasing them?

It is understood that emotions like anger and aggression need to be looked at more thoroughly before they are expressed, as they lead to hurting and offending others. But there is a tendency to suppress, control and bury all our emotions. Why do we feel that we cannot show our tears of sadness, our tears of sorrow to others? Why can't we express them at the moment they occur to the person who is causing it? The answer is always to say nothing, ignore how we feel, and it will all go away. But this is no longer good enough.

We know it is difficult but there is an art to it – there is a way of knowing. What do we need to do? We need to learn. Firstly, we ask ourselves if the offender crossed the emotional line. We need to decide what we will accept and what we will not accept. We need to learn ways of expressing ourselves that does not hurt or offend the other person but gets through to them and makes them hear and see our pain. We can then explain that their words and actions are not acceptable and that there are consequences and sacrifices being made by us that they should be aware of and that they should understand and that we are willing to listen to their side of the argument.

This process does not happen overnight. It takes practice. Sometimes we don't have the words to express how we feel or we lash out without thinking, but we may hear a song, someone on the radio or see someone on the tv who helps us articulate how we feel, go see a councillor, or talk to a friend but we need to learn ways to express our emotions so that no one gets hurt on both sides of the argument. We need to work on ways to express our emotions as best we can.

Now that we have defined our emotional line, the next step is to choose the best words to express how we feel. We need to reflect on our emotions that have built up over time which keep raising their dark head until we deal with them. No matter how big or small the emotional build up is, it will need to be let out and let go of but in a controlled, gentle, soft manner. We need to remember not to cross the emotional lines of both people but ensure these are always respected and honoured.

Emotions are not a bad thing – where would we be without emotions and feelings? We would be like robots. Is it not feelings that teaches us who we are, what we are about, what we can tolerate and what we cannot tolerate? How is that a bad thing? Emotions are not something bad but something beautiful. To be able to feel emotions is a genuine gift. Our emotions make us feel alive and human. We often hear people say, "Ooh, she/he is an emotional person but aren't they brave in showing their feelings as they are feeling them in that moment?"

Are they not owning their emotions? Are they not saying it as it is, not hiding how they really feel? But there is another line to draw once the emotions are expressed. There is a line to draw that we do not hurt the other person in the argument with our words or actions. Care is taken within the emotional outburst not to alienate or offend the other person. There is a level of control to be maintained. Remember that in explaining how we feel to another person, we draw an emotional line for them too.

Emotional healing may not happen in one conversation. It may take more than one conversation to discuss the depth of our emotions and their emotions, and these emotions may need to be revisited over a long period of time. The main thing we need to know is that there are consequences to emotional outbursts for all parties involved. These consequences include when and how we can express them, when and how we can allow them to surface, when and how long we can allow them time to heal, and when and how long we can allow our relationships to become stronger or let them go.

If someone is continually hurting us and we are overcome with pain and sorrow, we need to decide what is in our own best interests. We need to use the line we have drawn to protect ourselves. We should all learn to maintain our dignity. We should all learn to maintain our strength, our individuality and learn to be who we are. No one should be allowed to take that away from us. It is our divine right to be who we are. It is our divine gift to be ourselves, special and unique.

We are in charge of how we feel. No one has the right to intimidate, bully or make us feel uncomfortable. We need to learn to protect ourselves from their words, their actions and let them bounce off us. We need to learn not to let their words resonate in our heads. We need to let their words go. We need to learn to take action when they start affecting us emotionally. We do not allow the bully to take charge of our spirit, our mind, our heart. We do not allow them that power over us. We need to keep our mindset strong and learn to protect ourselves from the bully.

This is why emotions are so important they are like traffic lights – green for acceptable, amber for stop and examine, and red for danger. We need to own our emotions. No one should be allowed to treat us badly or hurt us. We need to stand up and be brave. Remember our emotions are the triggers that keep us healthy. They are the warning to us where to draw the line and that no one should be able to cross it, and in return, we will not cross their emotional line either.

We need to understand that emotions are part of our identity and are part of who we are. We are so delicate, so fragile and most of all, we are so human. We need to protect ourselves but if we bury our emotions, we bury our warning system, we bury our protection.

Let us teach ourselves to draw our emotional line that no one should cross or even want to cross, and we will reciprocate. Let us teach ourselves to express and vocalise our emotions in peace and harmony. Finally, we need to pass this teaching onto our children from a very young age to protect them and their children.

CHAPTER 37

Self-esteem

Say to yourself:

> I have a right to be here.
>
> I have my own uniqueness to offer.
>
> I am a special person.
>
> I have a value that is priceless.
>
> I am equal to everyone else.

Good self-esteem means that we know our worth, we value ourselves. Low self-esteem means we don't know our own worth. What happens if we change these negative assumptions to positive affirmations? We can change our lives.

The law of attraction really does work. Our thoughts have a positive charge and the universe picks up this charge. Sending out a positive charge means receiving a positive outcome. Sending a negative charge means receiving a negative outcome. It is that simple.

By breaking the negative opinions of ourselves, we can change. We can change how we think about ourselves. We can change how we feel about ourselves. We can change how we react to others. Instead of being full of anxiety and overloaded with negativity, we can learn to control it by filling our thoughts with only positive thoughts, ideas and opinions.

Instead of releasing a whole load of negative emotions and frustrations, we stay in the moment, acknowledging that we feel anxious, but we release it up to the universe and change our thought patterns to only positive ones. We don't allow our thoughts to control us, we control our thoughts. We switch the channel.

If we can think positively, feel positive, act positively and get positive reassurance from our family, peers and friends, we can change how we feel about ourselves. It is all about our belief, our trust, our confidence in our inner abilities to achieve our goals and our ability to keep trying and never giving up on our dreams and visions for a better life.

We have the right to have a good quality life. We have the right to have an easy life. We have the right to feel good about ourselves on the good days as well as on the bad days. By balancing our thoughts and by raising our self-esteem, we can change the lows into a balanced healthy feeling about ourselves.

Our own good, balanced self-esteem is all about loving ourselves, being comfortable with ourselves and being true to ourselves any time, any place or anywhere.

CHAPTER 38

Don't forget to laugh

Why do we forget to laugh when the greatest alternative medicine known to man is laughter? It warms and heals every cell, proton, electron, and neutron in our bodies. It kills all sadness, loneliness, and emptiness. Laughter is a gift. Laughter is a grace. Laughter is a present from the universe.

The ability to laugh heals all wounds and all pain. It makes our whole day richer. The ability to laugh can turn any argument into a manageable conversation where solutions can be found, and relationships can be strengthened and revived.

The ability to laugh turns any negative situation around into a buzzing frenzy of lightness and fun. Laughter is like bubbles of champagne dancing in the glass of life. Laughter is an essential tool in the toolbox of life because if we need to fix things or make changes in our lives that are difficult, laughter helps us make all those changes easier because laughter is as infectious as a fire spreading through a dry wood on a blistering hot summer's day.

Laughter when it erupts, catches hold and ignites the air with its roaring sound, burning through the atmosphere like a blazing inferno out of control, alive, wild and free. Nothing can dampen its force once the laughter crackles from the person or crowd, positivity ignites throughout the room like a cracking firework exploding on New Year's Eve. We all feel alive and vibrant inside. We all feel like dancing to the tune of life.

Laughter is medicine for the soul and spirit. Laughter makes the heart pump the blood of life through our veins and arteries making our emotions happily circulate to the rapid beat of life's drum, pulsating and dancing in a frenzy of joy and fulfilment. When is the last time you had a good laugh? Let's spread more laughter and cheer around us because life is just too short.

Share a laugh with someone today.

Please Review

Dear Reader,
If you enjoyed this book, would you kindly post a short review on Amazon or whatever platform you purchased the book from? Your feedback will make all the difference to getting the word out about this book.

To leave a review on Amazon, type in the book title. When you have found it and go to the book page, please scroll to the bottom of the page to where it says 'Write a Review' and then submit your review.

Thank you in advance.

Printed in Poland
by Amazon Fulfillment
Poland Sp. z o.o., Wrocław